Home Apothecary

BY

BENEDICT & AMELIA
WELLS

The content of this book is for general informational purposes only. Each person's physical, emotional, and spiritual condition is unique. The instruction in this book is not meant to be used, nor should it be used, to diagnose or treat any medical condition or to replace the services of your physician or other healthcare provider. The advice and strategies contained in the book may not be suitable for all readers. Please consult your healthcare provider for any questions that you may have about your own medical situation. Neither the author, publisher, nor any of their employees or representatives guarantees the accuracy of information in this book or its usefulness to a particular reader, nor are they responsible for any damage or negative consequence that may result from any treatment, action taken, or inaction by any person reading or following the information in this book.

ISBN:

Printed in the United States of America

TABLE OF CONTENTS

RECIPE LIST

CHAPTER 4

EVERYDAY WELLNESS AND FIRST AID

FIRST AID ESSENTIALS: QUICK HERBAL SOLUTIONS

EVERYDAY WELLNESS: BOOSTING IMMUNITY NATURALLY

HERBAL TEAS FOR COMMON AILMENTS

TINCTURES AND TONICS FOR ENERGY AND VITALITY

GUT HEALTH AND DIGESTION SUPPORT

EYE HEALTH AND VISION SUPPORT

SUPPORTING LIVER AND KIDNEY HEALTH NATURALLY

HERBAL APPROACHES TO CARDIOVASCULAR WELLNESS

CHILDREN'S HEALTH: SAFE REMEDIES FOR LITTLE ONES

SENIOR WELLNESS: HERBAL SUPPORT FOR AGING GRACEFULLY

PREGNANCY AND POSTPARTUM: HERBAL SUPPORT FOR MOTHERS

CHAPTER 7
CULINARY AND HOUSEHOLD APPLICATIONS

COOKING WITH MEDICINAL HERBS: FLAVOR MEETS WELLNESS

HERBAL INFUSIONS AND DECOCTIONS FOR HEALTHIER MEALS

ZERO WASTE PRACTICES: REDUCING YOUR ENVIRONMENTAL FOOTPRINT

ADAPTING RECIPES FOR DIETARY SENSITIVITIES

CHAPTER 8
SUSTAINABLE AND HEALTHY HOME SOLUTIONS

CREATING A CHEMICAL-FREE HOME CLEANING KIT

HERBAL PEST REPELLENTS: KEEPING YOUR HOME CRITTER-FREE

NATURAL AIR FRESHENERS: BREATHING EASY AT HOME

CRAFTING HERBAL LAUNDRY SOLUTIONS FOR SENSITIVE SKIN

ECO-FRIENDLY DISH AND SURFACE CLEANERS

INTRODUCTION

In a small, sunlit kitchen at the edge of town, jars line the shelves—amber, cobalt, and clear glass vessels holding dried flowers, roots, and leaves. Calendula petals catch the light like golden coins. A muslin bag filled with chamomile rests near a small mortar and pestle, and a kettle hums in the background. This is not a scene from a bygone era—it's happening right now in homes all over the world. Quietly, steadily, a revival is unfolding. People are reclaiming the simple act of crafting their own medicine—rooted in plants, guided by wisdom, and stirred by a desire for something more grounded, more intentional, and more real.

My own path to herbalism didn't start in a classroom. It began with curiosity and a deep need for change. I was tired of reading labels I couldn't pronounce, managing symptoms instead of addressing causes, and feeling disconnected from the care I was giving my family. What began with a single cup of lemon balm tea on a stressful night soon became an exploration into tinctures, salves, infused oils, and seasonal rituals that helped us feel better, sleep deeper, and live with more peace and confidence.

The more I learned, the more I remembered stories from my great-grandmother, who boiled wild plants for cough syrup, or neighbors who handed out elderberry syrup when school colds hit. I saw how herbalism wasn't about chasing trends. It was about remembering what we've always known. Every culture on earth has its own herbal tradition. These practices were born from observation, passed down through hands and voices, and kept alive through daily use. This knowledge is still alive—it just needs a place to grow.

A **home apothecary** is that place. It's your kitchen, your garden, your windowsill, your pantry. It's the cupboard where you keep dried herbs and the shelf where your labeled tinctures live. It's where healing becomes personal. Unlike commercial products that offer blanket solutions, your apothecary supports your unique body, your environment, and your values. Whether you're calming a child's fever with a tea blend or easing muscle tension with a homemade oil, each remedy becomes a conversation between you and the plants.

This book is a complete guide to creating your own home apothecary from the ground up. Inside, you'll find over 300 natural remedies for everyday wellness, seasonal support, and targeted care. From first aid salves to respiratory blends, immune tonics, and stress support formulas, each recipe is clear, approachable, and deeply rooted in traditional plant wisdom.

Part One lays the foundation. You'll learn how to set up your space, gather tools, safely work with herbs, and create personalized blends that match your family's needs. Part Two is your practical toolkit, organized by use and body system, age, and seasonal timing. Each chapter offers recipes, usage guidance, and optional variations—so you can adapt remedies to your preferences and needs.

Throughout this book, you'll also find reflections on sustainable living, gardening, eco-conscious choices, and the importance of stewardship. Herbalism isn't only about wellness—it's about building a relationship with the earth. The more we turn to plants for healing, the more we are reminded that we are part of something larger. A home apothecary supports both personal and planetary health.

What makes this book different is its blend of tradition and practicality. You don't need to be an herbalist to start—you just need the desire to care deeply. Whether you're making your first tea blend or customizing formulas for your whole family, you'll find the tools and confidence here to do it well.

This is more than a reference. It's an invitation—to reconnect with what matters, to heal with your hands, to listen to the wisdom of plants, and to remember that you already have everything you need to begin. Let's build your apothecary, one remedy at a time.

PART 1

LAYING THE GROUNDWORK: YOUR HOME APOTHECARY ESSENTIALS

Chapter 1

FOUNDATIONS OF THE HOME APOTHECARY

The cupboard smelled of earth and citrus. Jars lined the top shelf, each one labeled in a slanted, steady hand—comfrey, elderflower, fennel seed. A chipped mortar sat nearby, its bowl stained golden from years of grinding roots and bark. This wasn't a clinic. It was a kitchen. And it was where real healing happened.

Long before prescription bottles and urgent care, families reached for the plants they knew. They kept remedies close, tinctures in the pantry, salves by the bed, dried herbs hanging near the stove. Healing wasn't outsourced. It lived inside the home, passed down with recipes, rituals, and quiet confidence.

That knowledge has roots in nearly every culture. Whether it was a grandmother brewing peppermint tea for a child's bellyache or a village herbalist making poultices for burns, the practice of using plants as medicine was woven into daily life. It wasn't mystical. It was practical. And it worked.

This chapter lays the foundation for building that kind of relationship with plants again. You'll explore where the home apothecary came from—its role in ancient households, how it changed over time, and why it's finding its way back into modern homes. You'll see how plant-based remedies endured through centuries of change, carried by caregivers, healers, and home cooks alike.

There is a reason people are returning to this way of living. Not out of nostalgia, but because it makes sense. It's effective. It's accessible. And in many ways, it's the most natural thing you can do for your body, your family, and your home.

The home apothecary is more than a shelf of jars. It's a way of thinking. A way of preparing. A way of reclaiming the role of healer in your own space—with confidence, clarity, and a deep respect for the plants that support you.

REDISCOVERING THE FORGOTTEN APOTHECARY

A carved wooden shelf once held more than decoration. It was the medicine cabinet, the pharmacy, the kitchen lab. Jars filled with dried thyme, crushed pomegranate peel, or powdered bark didn't carry expiration dates—they carried generations of trust. In early homes and villages, healing was not outsourced. It was a skill, a role, a responsibility passed down through observation and practice. These weren't mystical rituals. They were daily essentials.

Apothecaries formed the backbone of ancient healing systems. In Egypt, formulas were recorded on papyrus scrolls with ingredients like myrrh, frankincense, and honey. Their temples held herb gardens. Their priests were botanists, blending faith with function. In Greece, Hippocrates taught that food and herbs were both prevention and cure. Galen, a Roman physician, developed herbal compounds that would influence Western pharmacology for centuries. These weren't side notes in history—they were central to health systems that endured for millennia.

In those early cultures, apothecaries functioned as more than dispensaries. They were repositories of practical knowledge, spiritual belief, and scientific inquiry. Healers used trial and error, observation, and ancestral teachings to understand the body in relation to the natural world. They studied the effects of plants not just on symptoms but on the whole person—physical, emotional, and energetic. This was healthcare integrated into the fabric of daily life.

As time moved forward, the role of the apothecary evolved. In medieval Europe, they worked alongside physicians, often preparing their remedies and maintaining herbal gardens. Their shops became trusted hubs—smelling of dried herbs, beeswax, and vinegar tinctures. In colonial times, herbalists were midwives, caretakers, and often the only available source of medicine. They carried knowledge rooted in the land, informed by tradition, and adapted to the needs of their community.

Global herbalism followed its own rich threads. In India, Ayurveda systematized plant medicine thousands of years ago—recognizing individual constitutions and seasonal rhythms in its treatments. Traditional Chinese Medicine developed complex herb pairings and formulas still used worldwide. Indigenous communities across the Americas, Africa, and Australia passed healing knowledge orally, tuning their medicine to what grew nearby, with a reverence for nature that was as spiritual as it was practical. Across all traditions, the herbalist was someone who listened closely—to people, to plants, to place.

Even the word "apothecary" itself carries weight. It implies preparation with care, knowledge held in the hands, healing crafted from what's on hand. The apothecary did not separate wellness from daily life—it was part of cooking, gardening, gathering, and caregiving.

Today, most people hear the word and picture something old-fashioned or decorative. Apothecary jars have become aesthetic props. But their original meaning has depth. Before synthetic drugs were mass-produced, people relied on their gardens, their kitchens, and their senses. Lavender for rest. Garlic for immunity. Slippery elm for sore throats. These weren't exotic secrets—they were household staples.

Over time, with the rise of modern pharmacology and the industrialization of healthcare, the apothecary faded into the background. The transition brought many benefits—sterility, precision, access—but it also severed something. The intuitive, plant-based healing that once empowered individuals became specialized, commercialized, and in many cases, forgotten.

Still, the knowledge never disappeared. It lived quietly in gardens, in old notebooks, in the stories told by elders, in rituals passed from one generation to the next. And now, it's being remembered—not out of nostalgia, but because it works.

What you're reading is not alternative. It's original. The recipes in this book don't belong to one culture, and they don't require a professional title to use. They belong to anyone who wants to make medicine in their own kitchen, with their own hands. This is the medicine of observation, of common sense, of patient care.

To rediscover the apothecary is to remember a way of living that honored the intelligence of plants and the participation of people. It's a return to something shared across cultures, across centuries. And it's never been more relevant than it is now.

THE DECLINE AND INDUSTRIAL DISCONNECTION

The shift didn't happen all at once. It crept in through glass bottles, factory labels, and brightly colored pills that promised relief without effort. One generation reached for their herb cupboard; the next reached for over-the-counter tablets. Convenience arrived quickly, and with it, a gradual silence fell over the home apothecary.

The Industrial Revolution brought sweeping changes to every corner of life, and medicine was no exception. Laboratories replaced kitchens. Standardized pills replaced handmade remedies. Extracts were separated from their plants and turned into compounds with long names and longer shelf lives. Healing became a product—measured, packaged, and sold on a shelf far removed from the garden or forest where it began.

As the pharmaceutical industry expanded, the collective memory of herbalism began to fade. What once lived in everyday rituals—steeping teas, preparing poultices, drying herbs near the fire—was now labeled outdated or unsanitary. Mass production offered speed and uniformity, but it also created distance. Distance from plants. Distance from the body's signals. Distance from self-trust.

Families who once passed down their healing knowledge through stories, gestures, and shared meals began to rely on prescriptions and instruction sheets. The role of the home healer was outsourced. The kitchen stopped being a place for medicine-making and became a staging ground for pre-packaged solutions.

The modern medical model advanced in many important ways. It brought surgical precision, emergency interventions, and scientific breakthroughs that saved lives. But in focusing on disease management, it often left little space for prevention, nourishment, and the slower wisdom of the plants. The patient became a passive recipient rather than an active participant.

What was lost in this shift wasn't just herbal knowledge—it was the confidence to care for ourselves. The rhythms of seasonal living, the observation of subtle changes, the belief that wellness starts with daily habits—all of it dulled in the bright glare of efficiency.

Still, the roots of that older wisdom remain. They show up in a grandmother's tea blend, in the instinct to reach for honey and lemon during a cold, in the curiosity sparked when someone smells lavender and feels something soften. The knowledge never disappeared. It waited. And now, it's ready to return.

HERBAL WISDOM ACROSS CONTINENTS

Plant medicine traveled across mountains, oceans, and deserts long before shipping containers and customs declarations. Seeds moved in the pockets of migrants. Remedies crossed borders with traders, healers, and colonizers alike. Over centuries, a global web of herbal knowledge formed—interwoven through trade routes, adaptation, and survival.

Despite the differences in language, climate, and culture, common threads appear in traditional healing systems around the world. Bitters for digestion. Roots for stamina. Flowers for calming the mind. Across continents, people discovered similar truths by observing the plants around them and listening to the body's response. These shared discoveries weren't coincidence. They were evidence of what works.

Turmeric, long prized in Indian Ayurvedic medicine for its anti-inflammatory and digestive properties, became a global staple through spice routes. Chamomile, native to Europe and used for sleep, skin, and digestion, now grows in gardens across the world. Mesoamerican cultures revered cacao not just as food but as heart medicine—warming, stimulating, and sacred. Ginger traveled from Asia to the Caribbean, where it became both culinary and medicinal. These plants crossed borders and found new homes without losing their purpose.

Local traditions adapted to local needs. Where one community relied on nettles, another used moringa. Where reishi mushrooms were used to calm the spirit in Traditional Chinese Medicine, North American tribes turned to skullcap. The form varied, but the intent remained: support the body's innate ability to heal.

What endured through colonization, displacement, and cultural suppression was the resilience of people and plants. Herbal traditions survived not because they were fashionable, but because they were essential. Passed down quietly in kitchens and forest walks, they held their ground.

Today's home apothecary doesn't begin from scratch—it draws from centuries of shared wisdom that belongs to everyone willing to learn, respect, and carry it forward.

THE MODERN REVIVAL OF THE HOME APOTHECARY

The jars are coming back. Not just as décor, but as daily tools. On kitchen counters and windowsills, people are once again filling glass vessels with oils, herbs, roots, and resins. Calendula blooms in backyard gardens. Elderberry syrup simmers on stovetops. Tinctures steep beside laptops. The home apothecary is no longer a relic—it's returning, freshly alive and deeply relevant.

There's a reason this revival is happening now. Many are reevaluating their relationship with health. The shelves lined with chemical-laden products, the long ingredient lists, the side effects, the costs—it all feels disconnected. In that gap, a quiet question rises: what did people do before all this?

The answer leads back to the plants. To hands-on remedies made with intention and simplicity. To self-trust and sustainability. This movement is about regaining agency—knowing how to soothe a sore throat, support a child's immunity, or ease anxiety without needing a prescription every time. It's not about rejecting modern medicine. It's about expanding the options.

People want medicine that makes sense. They want ingredients they can pronounce and harvest themselves. They want solutions that don't pollute their homes or their bodies. And they're finding them in herbalism.

From urban balconies to rural homesteads, this resurgence shows up in many forms. Farmers markets now sell dried herbs alongside produce. Online courses teach everything from foraging to formulation. Social media is full of makers sharing how to turn kitchen herbs into healing salves. Bookshelves are filling with guides on teas, tinctures, and tonics—just like this one.

This isn't a wellness trend chasing aesthetics. It's a return to something people forgot they could do. Herbal medicine isn't niche or fringe. It has always been here, waiting for its place back in the home.

You don't need to live off-grid or grow all your own herbs to take part. You only need a bit of space, a few jars, and the curiosity to start. The moment you dry your own chamomile or brew your own immunity tea, you step into a tradition far older than any pharmacy. This is how it begins—with one remedy, one ritual, and the quiet confidence that you already belong here.

REFLECTION: RECLAIMING YOUR HERBAL STORY

Pause for a moment.

Think back to a time when healing felt simple. Maybe it was a warm mug of ginger tea when you had a cold. A clove tucked between the cheek and gum for a toothache. Maybe it was the smell of eucalyptus in a bowl of steam, or the way your grandmother rubbed something from a jar onto your chest before bed.

These memories aren't random—they're roots. Threads of herbal wisdom passed down through touch, scent, and instinct.

Take a moment to reflect:

- What did healing look like in your family?
- What stories or remedies do you remember?
- What plants or smells bring you comfort?

Now picture your own healing space. What herbs would be on your shelf? What tools would live beside them? What would it feel like to reach for something you made, with your hands, for your body or someone you love?

There's no perfect starting point—just a willingness to remember and begin. Each remedy you create adds a new layer to your herbal story.

You are not starting from scratch.

You are returning to something ancient inside you.

Chapter 2

CRAFTING YOUR APOTHECARY TOOLKIT

Steam curls from a mug of steeping herbs as sunlight spills across the countertop. Glass jars line open shelves, each filled with leaves, roots, berries, or flowers—labeled neatly, worn with use. A small mortar sits nearby, still dusted with dried chamomile. This space hums with intention. It's not a laboratory. It's not a trend. It's a living extension of your care, your knowledge, and your desire to work with the plants that support your health.

This chapter marks the shift from learning into doing. The foundation has been laid—now comes the hands-on work of building your own apothecary. Whether you have an entire pantry to dedicate or a single shelf in your kitchen, this space becomes a reflection of your values and wellness needs. It is where herbs are stored, infused, blended, and transformed. It is where healing begins with your own two hands.

There's no one right way to set up a home apothecary. What matters is intention, clarity, and consistency. Some people begin with a few jars and build over time. Others start with a full setup. Either way, it helps to begin with a clear understanding of what you need and why.

This chapter will walk you through every essential piece: organizing your space, choosing your tools, sourcing quality herbs, growing a few reliable favorites, and safely storing and labeling everything you make. Whether your goal is to create a simple tea station or a full-spectrum healing kitchen, you'll learn how to approach this process with structure and care.

The apothecary you create will grow with you. It doesn't need to be perfect. It just needs to be functional, safe, and inspiring enough to keep your hands in the herbs and your focus on your health. You're not just collecting supplies—you're building a practice. One that nourishes, teaches, and quietly transforms the way you care for yourself and others. Let's begin.

ESSENTIAL PREPARATIONS FOR YOUR APOTHECARY JOURNEY

Building a home apothecary begins with clarity, not clutter. Before gathering tools, jars, or herbs, take a moment to understand why you're creating this space. Herbalism is not about having everything. It's about having what you need, knowing how to use it, and being consistent in your practice.

Start with a few simple questions. What are your current health goals? Are you building this apothecary to support immunity, improve sleep, reduce stress, ease digestion, or care for your children's wellness naturally? Maybe you're managing chronic inflammation, hormonal shifts, or simply want a safer, cleaner home environment. Write down a list of areas you'd like to support—personally or for your household. This becomes your apothecary blueprint.

Once you've named your priorities, sketch a basic outline of what a functional space would look like for you. A shelf in your kitchen? A drawer in your bathroom? A small cart that can be rolled between rooms? This doesn't require a full renovation. Many people start with a basket, a single box, or one pantry shelf. What matters is consistency and accessibility. If your herbs and tools are easy to reach, you'll use them more often.

Organize your space with both practicality and inspiration in mind. Jars should be clearly labeled, not just with the name of the herb but also its part (leaf, root, flower), date of purchase or harvest, and source. Use waterproof labels or hang simple handwritten tags with twine. Group herbs by category—digestive, immune, sleep—or by use frequency. Daily-use items should be front and center. Seasonal or specialty items can be stored away but easily accessed.

Beauty plays a role, too. A well-arranged shelf invites daily interaction. A cluttered or chaotic drawer makes you avoid it. Choose clear glass jars for visibility, use wooden trays or baskets to group like items, and display dried bundles or botanical art nearby. These small touches turn your apothecary into a creative, calming space.

Now, let's talk about tools. A basic apothecary doesn't require expensive equipment. Start with a **mortar and pestle** for grinding dried herbs or use a clean coffee grinder. You'll also need **cheesecloth or muslin bags** for straining infusions and tinctures, and **fine mesh strainers** or **funnel filters** for oils and syrups. Keep a collection of **glass jars** in various sizes—preferably amber or cobalt for light protection. A **digital scale** with gram precision is helpful when following or recording exact formulations. Other helpful items include **measuring spoons, a stainless-steel saucepan, dropper bottles, labels**, and **a dedicated cutting board** for roots and resins.

If you're on a budget, look at what you already have. A clean cotton dish towel can substitute for straining. Reuse jam jars or spice containers. Ask friends or family for any extra canning supplies. Over time, as your practice deepens, you'll refine and upgrade what you use most.

Sourcing herbs requires attention and care. Quality matters. The effectiveness of your remedies depends on the freshness, purity, and correct identification of the plant. Two of the most respected sources in the U.S. are **Mountain Rose Herbs** and **Frontier Co-op**—both of which offer organic, sustainably harvested options and detailed profiles for each plant. You can also look for regional herb farms, community-supported herbal shares, or local herb shops where you can see and smell what you're buying.

Buying in bulk is cost-effective, but only buy what you'll use in the next 6-12 months. Herbs lose potency with time, especially if exposed to light, heat, or moisture. For rare or specialty herbs, work with trusted herbalists or growers who can ensure proper identification and harvesting practices.

If you want even more control over quality and cost, grow your own. Starting with a few easy plants—like **calendula**, **peppermint**, **chamomile**, or **lemon balm**—gives you fresh, organic material right outside your door. This will be covered in detail in the next section, but even a few potted plants can provide more than you think.

As your collection grows, so does the need for order. Use a **notebook or digital spreadsheet** to track what you've made, what you've used, and what needs to be replenished. Include harvest or purchase dates, notes on how the remedy worked, and any observations about changes in taste, color, or potency. This recordkeeping not only saves time—it builds your confidence and gives you data to work from.

Integrating organization and beauty isn't just about aesthetics—it supports your consistency. A well-kept apothecary becomes part of your daily rhythm. You'll know exactly where your elderberry is when the first sniffle hits. Your calendula oil won't be lost in the back of a cupboard. And your tinctures will be labeled clearly enough to use and share without hesitation.

Even small rituals around your apothecary matter. Light a candle when making remedies. Set your jars in the sun to infuse with warmth and intention. Open a window to let in fresh air as you mix and pour. These practices aren't about performance. They're about care—and care increases effectiveness.

Before moving forward, let's address safety. Herbalism is a powerful form of self-care, and with that comes responsibility. Not every herb is safe for every person or situation. Some interact with medications. Others require specific preparation methods. Always consult reliable references—books by clinical herbalists, vetted herbal databases, or trusted teachers. Don't rely on unverified internet sources. Keep a few go-to safety guides on your shelf and refer to them often.

If you're making remedies for others, especially children, pregnant individuals, or elders, do a second layer of research. Record keeping helps here, too. Note which herbs you've used in each product, the ratios, and any relevant cautions. This also helps if you're ever asked to repeat a remedy—or explain it.

In some regions, selling homemade herbal products requires legal steps: cottage food laws, product labeling standards, or licenses. Even if you're only crafting for personal use, it's wise to stay informed about the rules in your area. Herbalism thrives when it's practiced responsibly.

What you're building is more than a shelf of jars. It's a system of care, a support network built from leaves and roots and glass. With a small amount of planning, the right tools, and thoughtful sourcing, your apothecary becomes a daily resource—organized, beautiful, and ready to serve. Whether you're steeping a cup of tea or blending a balm, this space becomes a container for skill, healing, and intention. It's where knowledge turns into practice. And where practice becomes daily care.

CULTIVATING HERBAL MEDICINES IN YOUR BACKYARD

The scent of crushed peppermint on your fingertips, the soft rustle of calendula petals in the morning breeze, the quiet satisfaction of watching your lavender bloom—this is herbal medicine in its most accessible form. Whether you have a large backyard or a single sunny balcony, you have everything needed to grow healing right where you live.

Herbalism begins with the plants themselves. Working with herbs becomes far more intimate when you've grown them from seed or starter. You learn their preferences. You notice how they change with the seasons. You witness the conditions that bring out their potency and their beauty. This connection shapes not just how you use herbs, but how you care for them, and ultimately, how they care for you.

Start with a few reliable allies. *Chamomile* is both calming and resilient, thriving in pots or raised beds and offering a steady harvest of small, daisy-like flowers. *Peppermint* grows quickly and spreads easily, making it ideal for container growing to keep it contained. *Calendula* produces bright orange and yellow blooms with powerful skin-healing properties and continues to flower throughout the growing season. *Lavender* prefers full sun and dry soil and rewards your care with aromatic blossoms perfect for teas, sachets, and infusions.

Choose a growing area that receives at least six hours of sunlight a day. Most culinary and medicinal herbs thrive in bright light. Prepare your soil by loosening it deeply and mixing in compost. If your space is limited or your soil is poor, use large containers with drainage holes and a high-quality organic potting mix. Herbs generally prefer soil that drains well and won’t stay soggy between waterings.

Give your plants room to breathe. Overcrowding reduces airflow and invites mildew or pests. Follow spacing instructions for each herb, allowing enough room for roots to spread and foliage to develop. Place taller herbs like echinacea or lemon balm toward the back of your bed or container layout, with shorter ones like thyme or chamomile near the front or edges.

Watering should be consistent but moderate. Most herbs dislike wet feet. Water early in the day so leaves can dry in the sun, reducing fungal risks. During hot spells or peak summer growth, container herbs may need daily watering, while those in the ground often require less frequent attention.

Pest control in an herbal garden starts with observation. Check under leaves regularly for aphids or caterpillars. Invite beneficial insects like ladybugs and lacewings by planting diversity. Sprinkle crushed eggshells around your plants to deter slugs. A light spray made of diluted neem oil or castile soap and water can help manage soft-bodied pests without harming the plants. Avoid harsh chemical treatments that could compromise the medicinal quality of your herbs.

Plant combinations thoughtfully. Companion planting helps create balance and reduces maintenance. Basil grows well alongside tomatoes and repels aphids. Calendula supports pollinators and adds cheer to any border. Mint helps deter ants but spreads aggressively—best kept in pots near garden perimeters.

Even with limited space or harsh climates, indoor growing works well with the right setup. A sunny windowsill can host potted rosemary, thyme, or chives. If light is limited, full spectrum grow lights allow you to cultivate medicinal herbs in colder months or shaded apartments. Water with care, and rotate pots weekly to encourage even growth.

Tending your garden offers more than ingredients for your remedies. It becomes a form of therapy. Pulling weeds clears the mind. Watching a seed germinate brings a quiet sense of accomplishment. Spending time with the plants you'll later brew or bottle deepens your understanding of how healing starts—with attention, presence, and small, consistent acts of care.

Growing your own herbs offers long-term savings. A single packet of seeds costs less than a jar of dried herbs and can yield enough to stock your home apothecary for the year. Even better, you know the exact source, treatment, and harvest date of each plant. There's no need to wonder about quality when you've cultivated it yourself.

Herbal gardening also supports sustainable living. Reducing reliance on shipping and packaging, reusing containers, and composting plant waste all contribute to a low-waste practice. Even your trimmings and leftovers can be returned to the soil as mulch or compost, continuing the cycle of nourishment.

As you build your garden, keep notes. Record which plants thrive in your space, which ones need more attention, and how you use each harvest. These records become part of your herbal education. They allow you to plan better each season and refine your growing practice as your apothecary expands.

Whether you're harvesting lavender for sleep sachets, gathering lemon balm for stress teas, or drying calendula petals to infuse in oil, you'll begin to see your plants not just as ingredients—but as partners in care. A homegrown apothecary starts with a single pot, a single season, and the decision to grow with purpose. Healing, after all, begins at home—and often, right in the dirt.

HARVESTING, STORING, AND USING HERBAL MEDICINE

The moment you clip your first calendula flower or pull a fragrant root from the soil, the transformation begins. Harvesting is not just a step in herbal preparation—it's the moment your relationship with the plant becomes tangible. Timing, method, and intention all shape the potency of your remedies. The more you pay attention, the more effective your medicine becomes.

Each part of a plant has its own harvest window. **Leaves** are best collected in the morning after the dew has evaporated but before the sun is too strong. This helps preserve their oils and vitality. Choose healthy, vibrant leaves, free from spots or pests. Plants like lemon balm, mint, and nettle offer multiple leaf harvests throughout the season when trimmed properly.

Flowers should be gathered just after they open, when their color and scent are strongest. Chamomile, calendula, and lavender respond well to regular picking, which encourages more blooms. Use clean scissors or fingers to snip them at the base and handle gently to preserve their delicate structures.

Roots are typically harvested in the fall, after the plant's energy has returned underground. This is when medicinal compounds are most concentrated. Dandelion, burdock, and echinacea roots can be carefully dug with a trowel, rinsed well, and chopped before drying. For biennials like mullein or burdock, wait until the end of their first growing season.

Work in alignment with the seasons. Spring and early summer are ideal for harvesting greens and flowers. Fall is best for roots and barks. Avoid harvesting during extreme weather, after rainfall, or from plants that are stressed or diseased. Always leave some behind—both to honor the plant and to allow regrowth for future seasons.

Once you've harvested, the next step is preservation. For most herbs, **air-drying** is the simplest and most traditional method. Bundle small groups of stems and hang them upside down in a well-ventilated, shaded area. You can also use **drying racks**, especially for flowers or loose leaves. Avoid plastic containers or direct sunlight, which can cause mold or degrade volatile oils.

For faster drying, a **dehydrator** with a low-temperature setting (95-115Â°F or 35-46Â°C) can help retain color and aroma. Spread herbs in a single layer and check them daily. Once fully dry, they should crumble easily between your fingers with no moisture left.

Some herbs—like basil, rosemary, or chives—can also be preserved by **freezing**. Blend them with a neutral oil like olive oil and pour into ice cube trays. Once frozen, transfer cubes to labeled freezer bags. This method preserves color and flavor well for culinary or topical use.

Once dried or frozen, store herbs in **glass jars with tight-fitting lids**—preferably amber or cobalt to protect from light. Keep them in a cool, dark place like a cabinet or pantry. Avoid plastic containers, as they may absorb oils or leach chemicals over time. Label each jar clearly with the plant name, part used, date harvested, and origin (e.g., "Homegrown peppermint leaf - July 2025-Backyard Garden").

For herbs you've purchased, transfer them from paper or plastic bags into jars as soon as possible. Note the supplier and date received. Even commercially dried herbs lose potency over time. Aim to use most herbs within one year, though some roots and barks retain strength longer.

Once your herbs are stored, you're ready to begin using them. Start with **infusions**, which are simply strong teas. Pour boiling water over dried leaves or flowers, cover, and steep for 15-30 minutes—or longer for medicinal strength. This method works well for nettle, lemon balm, and red raspberry leaf.

Decoctions are used for tougher parts like roots, bark, or seeds. Simmer herbs gently in water for 20-40 minutes to extract their compounds. Ginger, licorice, and dandelion root respond well to this method.

Tinctures involve soaking herbs in alcohol (usually vodka or brandy) for 4-6 weeks. This extracts and preserves the active compounds, creating a potent remedy that lasts for years. You'll find detailed instructions for this in a later chapter.

Salves and oils are made by infusing herbs into oil and then blending with beeswax or another base. These are ideal for skin support, muscle soreness, or minor wounds—again, full tutorials are coming soon.

Even as you begin to craft your first preparations, track everything. Keep a dedicated notebook, binder, or digital log with notes for each harvest, recipe, and outcome. Record the herb, the date, how it was prepared, and how it worked. These records become your herbal memory. They help you refine your methods, remember what you've made, and pass knowledge along with confidence.

Herbs integrate most easily into daily routines when they're visible, ready to use, and connected to your actual needs. Start your morning with a nourishing infusion. Keep a jar of lemon balm glycerite near your tea kettle. Add fresh herbs to your cooking. Drop a lavender sachet in your pillowcase. These small acts bring your apothecary to life—not just as a storage space, but as a rhythm of care.

A well-tended shelf of herbal remedies is more than practical. It's personal. Every jar holds not just a plant, but a decision—a choice to be present, informed, and proactive about your wellness. Over time, your apothecary becomes a map of what your body needed, how it responded, and what you learned.

Your apothecary is now a living library of your healing journey—each leaf harvested, each remedy made, a page written in wisdom and care.

REFLECTION: ALIGNING WITH YOUR HERBAL PATH

Take a breath and look at what you've begun to build. Whether your apothecary is a single windowsill, or a cabinet filled with jars, this space now reflects your decision to care differently—more intentionally, more naturally, and with your hands involved in the process.

What health areas feel most important to you right now? Maybe you're focused on calming stress, improving digestion, supporting your immune system, or caring for your family in more natural ways. Write them down. Let them guide what you grow, gather, and prepare.

Are there specific herbs you feel drawn to? Sometimes the connection is practical—like needing chamomile for sleep. Other times, it's intuitive. Maybe you've always loved the smell of lavender, or your grandmother used to grow mint in her garden. Follow that spark. Curiosity is often your first teacher.

Now, choose one small habit to begin this week. Brew a daily herbal tea. Organize your jars. Make your first infusion. It doesn't need to be perfect—it just needs to be consistent.

Finally, give your apothecary space a name if you'd like. Say a blessing over it. Light a candle. Let this be more than storage—it's a sacred corner of your home where healing lives. And it belongs to you.

You now have the space, tools, and mindset to begin working with herbs in a practical, grounded way. Your apothecary is no longer an idea—it's a functional part of your home and your wellness practice. With your shelves stocked, your tools in place, and your intentions set, you're ready to begin the next phase of herbal living.

But before diving into formulas and advanced remedies, it's essential to learn how to use herbs wisely and safely. Just like food or medicine, herbs interact with the body in specific ways. Understanding dosage, preparation methods, and contraindications ensures that your care is both effective and responsible.

Chapter 3

SAFE AND EFFECTIVE HERBAL PRACTICES

The kettle hisses softly. A scoop of dried elderberries falls into a glass jar, followed by cinnamon, cloves, and a few slices of fresh ginger. As the hot water pours, the aroma begins to rise—sharp, sweet, and familiar. There's comfort in making your own medicine, but there's also a responsibility.

Herbs are powerful. A single plant can calm a child's anxiety, ease inflammation, or disrupt a prescription drug's effect. This is why herbalism must be practiced with knowledge and intention. It isn't about guessing or following trends. It's about understanding how to work with plants safely, so their benefits are used wisely—and their risks are avoided.

This chapter is your foundation for safe and effective use. You'll learn how to set up your workspace for clean, responsible preparation. You'll understand proper dosing—what's appropriate for teas versus tinctures, and how to adjust for children or sensitive individuals. You'll learn how to identify herbs accurately, and how to recognize potential allergies or sensitivities before they become problems.

You'll also explore how herbs interact with prescription medications and how to assess claims using both tradition and science. Each of these topics builds your confidence and your discernment.

You're not just blending teas or bottling tinctures. You're working with living medicine. This chapter ensures you do it with care, clarity, and wisdom. Let's begin.

SAFETY FIRST: HANDLING HERBAL MEDICINE WITH CARE

A clean, organized workspace is the foundation of safe herbal preparation. When you work with medicinal plants, you're handling substances that directly influence the body—internally and externally. The conditions in which you blend, steep, and bottle matter just as much as the ingredients themselves.

Start with your environment. Choose a workspace that is well-ventilated, well-lit, and free from distractions. A dedicated surface, even if small, should be wiped down thoroughly before and after each session. Avoid preparing herbal remedies near areas used for raw meat, strong cleaners, or perfumed products. If possible, store your apothecary tools in a separate container from kitchen cookware to avoid contamination.

Always sanitize your tools. Wash glass jars with hot, soapy water and rinse thoroughly. For tincture bottles, droppers, or oil infusers, use boiling water or a sanitizing rinse like diluted alcohol to ensure clean handling. Cutting boards and knives used for roots and barks should be designated for herbs only. Cross-use with food prep or cleaning products can compromise both potency and safety.

Some herbalists also use protective gear when working with potent or resinous plants. Gloves protect the skin from strong oils or allergens, especially when processing chili peppers, mustards, or sticky resins like pine or myrrh. Goggles are helpful when blending powders or working with airborne particles like dried calendula petals or powdered cayenne. A simple cotton mask reduces risk when handling herbs that may irritate the lungs or trigger allergies.

Not all herbs are gentle. Certain plants require extra caution or professional guidance. *Foxglove* (Digitalis purpurea), while historically used for heart conditions, contains cardiac glycosides that can be toxic even in small amounts. *Comfrey* (Symphytum officinale) is a popular wound-healing herb but contains pyrrolizidine alkaloids, which may damage the liver if used internally or over broken skin for extended periods. *Hemlock* (Conium maculatum) is extremely toxic and often mistaken for safe lookalikes like wild carrot or parsley. It is not an herb for home use under any circumstances.

Cross-contamination is another concern. If you're preparing multiple remedies at once, keep ingredients and tools separate until you're ready to clean between uses. Allergens can transfer easily—especially when working with common triggers like chamomile (a relative of ragweed), nettle, or cinnamon. Label everything clearly and consistently. Even if you know your herbs well, a guest or family member might not.

Assumptions can be dangerous in herbalism. Just because an herb is popular doesn't make it universally safe. *Elderberry* syrup is widely known for immune support, but using raw, unripe berries or leaves can cause nausea or worse due to cyanogenic glycosides. *Licorice root* is effective for adrenal support and coughs, but it can raise blood pressure if taken in large amounts over time. Always reference well-sourced herbal guides or consult with experienced herbalists when using a new plant.

Trustworthy resources matter. Avoid relying on social media posts or unverified blogs for dosage or preparation methods. Instead, lean on books written by trained herbalists, peer-reviewed research, and reputable herbal organizations. Some recommended authors and educators include Rosemary Gladstar, David Hoffman, and Aviva Romm, along with organizations like the American Herbalists Guild and the National Center for Complementary and Integrative Health (NCCIH).

Approaching herbal medicine with reverence means approaching it with responsibility. Your remedies are only as effective as the care you put into making them. Clean tools, clear labeling, and informed choices protect you and the people you serve.

Reflection Box

- What does your current workspace look like?
- Is it clean, quiet, and organized for safe herbal preparation?
- What tools need to be cleaned, replaced, or set aside for herbal use only?
- Could gloves, masks, or goggles help you handle certain herbs with more confidence?
- What habits can you create to ensure safety becomes second nature in your herbal practice?

UNDERSTANDING DOSAGES AND MEASUREMENTS

Dosage is where the art of herbalism meets responsibility. Plants contain active compounds that interact with the body in measurable ways. While herbal medicine is generally gentle and forgiving, quantity still matters. A remedy taken too weakly may be ineffective; taken too strongly, it may cause unwanted effects. The key is to find the right amount for the right person at the right time.

Each form of herbal preparation delivers a different level of potency. Understanding these differences helps you use herbs effectively and safely.

Teas and infusions are among the most accessible forms. A cup of chamomile tea made with one teaspoon of dried flowers steeped for 10 minutes offers a mild calming effect. Doubling the amount or steeping too long can lead to bitterness or even digestive discomfort in sensitive individuals. For more medicinal strength, use an infusion—typically one tablespoon of dried herb steeped in 1-2 cups of hot water for 30 minutes or more. Nettle and red raspberry leaf are commonly prepared this way to extract vitamins and minerals.

Tinctures are concentrated liquid extracts made with alcohol or glycerin. They offer stronger, faster absorption. A common echinacea tincture dose is 2-3 milliliters (about 60-90 drops) taken three times daily at the onset of cold symptoms. Tinctures should always be measured with a dropper or small dosing cup. The strength can vary depending on the plant-to-solvent ratio, so follow specific instructions for each formula.

Capsules and powders provide convenience but require consistency. Doses are often standardized—such as 500 mg of turmeric powder per capsule—but may still need adjustment based on body size or condition. Always verify the milligram content on labels, and avoid assuming that more capsules mean better results.

Accurate measurement tools are essential. Keep a **digital kitchen scale** for weighing dried herbs, especially when creating custom formulas. **Measuring spoons** help with standardizing tea and infusion quantities. **Glass droppers** and **small graduated cylinders** ensure precise tincture dosing. A **mortar and pestle** is helpful for crushing herbs evenly, especially when making capsules or salves.

Individual needs vary. A healthy adult may tolerate a full-strength tincture three times per day, while someone with a smaller body frame, compromised liver function, or multiple medications may need a lower dose. Start with the minimum effective amount and increase only if needed. Sensitivity differs person to person. Some may feel a noticeable effect from a mild tea; others may require a more concentrated preparation to experience results.

Dosing for children requires special care. Their bodies process compounds differently, and even gentle herbs must be used thoughtfully. One commonly used formula for children's dosing is Clark's Rule:

$$\textbf{(Weight of child in pounds} \div \textbf{150)} \times \textbf{adult dose}$$

So, if an adult dose is 3 mL of tincture and the child weighs 50 pounds, the dose would be about 1 mL.

Avoid giving internal herbal remedies to infants under 6 months without professional guidance. For children between 6 months and 2 years, teas or diluted glycerites are often preferred over alcohol-based tinctures. Always introduce herbs one at a time and monitor for allergic reactions such as rashes, fussiness, or digestive upset.

Elderly individuals may also require adjusted dosages due to changes in metabolism, sensitivity, or existing medical conditions. Start low and monitor closely. Herbs like hawthorn, ginkgo, and valerian can be supportive but should be balanced with attention to potential interactions with medications or chronic conditions.

Herbal dosing is not one-size-fits-all. It is both science and skill—built on careful observation, clear measurements, and the willingness to adjust based on response. Keeping notes in your herbal journal about how each herb affects you or your loved ones helps fine-tune your approach over time.

Herbs are powerful partners in wellness, and dosage is the language they speak. Learning how to measure wisely means working with your herbs—not just using them. Precision doesn't limit herbalism; it strengthens it. When you know how much to give, and when, your remedies become more effective, more trustworthy, and more aligned with care.

IDENTIFYING HERBS: A BEGINNER'S GUIDE

Correct plant identification is not optional—it's essential. A mistake in recognizing a plant could mean the difference between a healing cup of tea and a harmful reaction. Many useful herbs have lookalikes, and while some are benign, others are toxic. Every herbalist, no matter how new, needs to develop sharp eyes and a healthy respect for plant features.

Start with the basics: leaf shape, color, scent, and growth habits. These four characteristics are your entry points for reliable identification.

Leaf shape tells you a lot. Is the leaf rounded, pointed, lobed, or serrated? Chamomile leaves are fine and feathery, while plantain leaves are broad with visible vertical veins. Lavender has narrow, silvery leaves with a slight fuzz. Take time to study and compare shapes—both the individual leaf and how it grows on the stem.

Color is another clue. Most herbs are green, but the shade matters. Peppermint has a deep, rich green, while lemon balm leans toward a lighter, more yellow-toned green. Some herbs have purple tints on the stems or undersides. Color can also change as the plant matures or depending on growing conditions, so compare multiple specimens when possible.

Scent may be the most helpful identifier, especially for aromatic herbs. Crush a small leaf between your fingers. Does it release a strong smell? Basil, mint, and rosemary all give off distinct, unmistakable aromas. Scent can help distinguish lookalikes, especially among mints, which share similar leaf structures but vary dramatically in fragrance.

Growth habits include how a plant spreads, how tall it grows, and what kind of environment it prefers. Calendula grows in upright, bushy clumps, while creeping thyme hugs the ground. Yarrow has tall, feathery stalks topped with flat flower clusters. Observing where a plant grows—sun or shade, wet or dry soil—also supports proper ID.

Use multiple points of identification before harvesting or using a plant. Don't rely on a single feature. The best approach includes confirming at least three or four traits: shape, scent, color, and growing pattern.

Reliable tools help deepen your accuracy. **Field guides** with full-color photographs are a must-have. Choose ones specific to your region, as native species vary widely by climate and geography. Digital apps like *PlantSnap* or *Picture. This* allow you to take a photo and receive instant suggestions, but always double-check the result with a physical guide or cross-reference.

Creating your own **herbarium** is a hands-on way to learn. Press and dry leaves, tape them into a notebook, and label them with the plant's name, date found, location, and any notes on scent, use, or growing conditions. Over time, this builds your personal library of local herbs and strengthens your observation skills.

Start small. Get to know five or six herbs really well before expanding. Focus on ones that grow nearby or that you use often in your apothecary. Take your time. Herbal knowledge is built in layers—through sight, smell, touch, and memory.

Activity Box: Build Your Herbal Eye

Go on a herb identification walk in your neighborhood, garden, or a local park.

- ☐ Take photos of 3-5 different plants that catch your attention.
- ☐ Sketch one of the leaves in your journal—note the shape, size, and edge.
- ☐ Gently crush a leaf and record the scent.
- ☐ Use a field guide or app to identify each plant and write down its name and possible uses.
- ☐ Begin your herbarium with one dried and labeled sample.

Keep building this practice. Over time, your confidence will grow—and your herbal work will become not only safer, but far more connected to the living world around you.

ADDRESSING ALLERGIES AND SENSITIVITIES

Even gentle herbs can cause strong reactions in sensitive individuals. While most herbs are well-tolerated when used properly, allergies and sensitivities are real and should always be part of your safety considerations—especially when creating remedies for others.

Some plants are more likely to cause allergic responses than others. **Chamomile**, for example, is part of the Asteraceae family, which includes ragweed, daisies, and marigolds. People with ragweed allergies may experience reactions to chamomile ranging from mild itching to sneezing or skin irritation. **Yarrow**, **echinacea**, and **feverfew** are also in this plant family and can trigger similar responses.

Other common triggers include **cinnamon**, **clove**, **peppermint**, and **garlic**—not because they're inherently harmful, but because they contain strong essential oils that may irritate sensitive skin or mucous membranes, especially in concentrated forms like tinctures, salves, or essential oil blends.

When using a new herb, especially topically, do a **patch test**. Apply a small amount of the diluted preparation (such as an oil or salve) to the inside of your forearm or behind your ear. Wait 24 hours and monitor for signs like redness, itching, swelling, or discomfort. For internal use, start with a small dose and wait several hours before increasing, especially if you've had allergic reactions in the past.

Know the **red flags** of allergic or adverse responses:

- Rash, itching, or hives
- Swelling, especially around the face or throat

- Tingling or burning sensations on the skin or tongue
- Trouble breathing, coughing, or wheezing
- Digestive upset like nausea, cramping, or diarrhea

If any of these symptoms occur, stop using the herb immediately. In the case of respiratory distress or throat swelling, seek emergency medical attention.

If you or someone you're preparing for has known sensitivities, substitutions can keep herbal care accessible and safe. For immune support, astragalus is a gentle alternative to echinacea, especially for those who react to Asteraceae plants. Holy basil offers adaptogenic and respiratory benefits similar to mint, but with a lower risk of sensitivity. Instead of comfrey for wound healing, try calendula, which offers similar skin-soothing effects with a better safety profile for most users.

When crafting blends, limit the number of herbs at first. This makes it easier to identify which ingredient is responsible in case of a reaction. Record every ingredient used, including oils, waxes, and carrier bases. Natural does not always mean risk-free—each body responds differently.

If you're preparing remedies for children, elders, or those with asthma, autoimmune conditions, or multiple allergies, always err on the side of caution. Start with food herbs like ginger, fennel, lemon balm, or nettles, which tend to be better tolerated. And when in doubt, consult a trained herbalist or integrative health professional.

Checklist Box: Crafting Allergen-Free Remedies

☐ Check for known allergies to plant families (e.g., Asteraceae, Lamiaceae).

☐ Use patch testing before topical application.

☐ Introduce one new herb at a time.

☐ Document every ingredient used.

- ☐ Use food-grade herbs for higher tolerance.
- ☐ Keep remedies simple—2-3 herbs max for first-time blends.
- ☐ Substitute known irritants with gentler herbs when possible.
- ☐ Monitor symptoms closely after each use.
- ☐ Store remedies in clearly labeled containers.
- ☐ When preparing for others, always ask about allergies first.

Clear, attentive preparation keeps herbalism inclusive, safe, and trusted. Sensitivity doesn't have to mean avoidance—it simply calls for thoughtful crafting and a deep respect for individual needs.

BALANCING HERBAL REMEDIES WITH PRESCRIBED MEDICATIONS

Herbal remedies and pharmaceutical medications both have real effects on the body—and when combined without awareness, those effects can interfere with each other. This doesn't mean you must choose one or the other. It means you must be informed, attentive, and transparent.

Herb-drug interactions occur when a plant alters how a medication is absorbed, processed, or eliminated. This can either increase the drug's effect to a dangerous level or reduce its effectiveness altogether.

One of the most well-known examples is **St. John's Wort**, often used for mild depression and mood support. It speeds up the liver's detox pathways, which can cause certain medications to clear from the body too quickly making antidepressants, birth control pills, or blood thinners less effective. This interaction isn't subtle. In some cases, it can completely neutralize a prescription.

Garlic, taken in therapeutic amounts for heart health or cholesterol, can thin the blood. Combined with prescribed blood thinners like warfarin, it increases the risk of excessive bleeding. **Ginkgo biloba** can have a similar effect.

These aren't reasons to avoid herbs. They are reasons to respect them. The solution starts with open communication. Always tell your doctor or pharmacist if you are using or planning to use herbal remedies—especially if you're on long-term or high-risk prescriptions. Many healthcare professionals appreciate patients who are proactive and clear about their wellness routines.

Timing and spacing also play a role. Taking a medication and an herb at the same time may heighten the chance of interaction. In some cases, spacing them out by a few hours reduces the risk. Journaling your daily intake—what you take, when, and how you feel—can help identify patterns, benefits, or problems early.

If you're unsure about a specific combination, check reputable resources like the Memorial Sloan Kettering Integrative Medicine database or the National Institutes of Health (NIH) supplement fact sheets. These are trustworthy starting points to verify safety.

Herbalism and conventional medicine are not enemies. Informed choices allow both to work in harmony. Whether you are healing from illness, managing a chronic condition, or supporting overall wellness, your decisions matter—and so does the quality of your information.

When herbal remedies are chosen with care and used alongside medical treatment with clarity, they can complement and strengthen your overall health plan. There's wisdom in the plants, and there's wisdom in partnership.

Traditional herbal knowledge has stood the test of time, but today's herbalist also benefits from tools that our ancestors didn't have—namely, science. Modern research doesn't replace generational wisdom; it sharpens it. When used together, tradition and evidence form a more complete understanding of how plants work in the body.

Many herbs used for centuries are now supported by peer-reviewed studies. Echinacea, commonly used for immune support, has shown in controlled trials to reduce the duration and severity of colds when taken at the onset of symptoms. **Turmeric**, long used in Ayurvedic medicine for inflammation, contains curcumin—a compound now studied for its anti-inflammatory and antioxidant effects in conditions ranging from arthritis to metabolic syndrome.

Scientific research helps confirm what herbalists have practiced for generations. It also helps clarify dosage, standardize extracts, and uncover how certain compounds interact with the body. For example, studies on **valerian root** have helped validate its use for sleep support, and **peppermint oil** has been clinically evaluated for digestive discomfort such as irritable bowel syndrome.

To assess herbal claims, go beyond marketing. Terms like "clinically proven" or "ancient remedy" can be misleading without context. Look for studies published in **peer-reviewed journals**—those that involve controlled experiments, clearly defined results, and transparent methodologies.

Start with accessible, trustworthy databases:

- **PubMed** (pubmed.gov): A comprehensive archive of biomedical literature
- National Center for Complementary and Integrative Health (NCCIH)**: Offers fact sheets, safety profiles, and current research**
- **American Herbal Pharmacopoeia** and **HerbalGram** (by the American Botanical Council): Focused resources for in-depth plant monographs and clinical data

Avoid anecdotal-only sources or products that don't disclose ingredient amounts or sourcing. Transparency is key. The more you understand what's in your herbal remedy and how it's meant to work, the more confidently you can use it—or choose an alternative.

Using herbs based on both ancestral use and modern validation creates a balanced, informed approach. One honors lived experience, the other supports measurable outcomes. Both are valuable.

Your respect for both wisdom and science makes you a mindful herbalist. You're not choosing sides—you're building skill. This kind of discernment not only protects your health, but also deepens your trust in the remedies you make, use, and share.

PART 2

HOME REMEDIES FOR EVERYONE

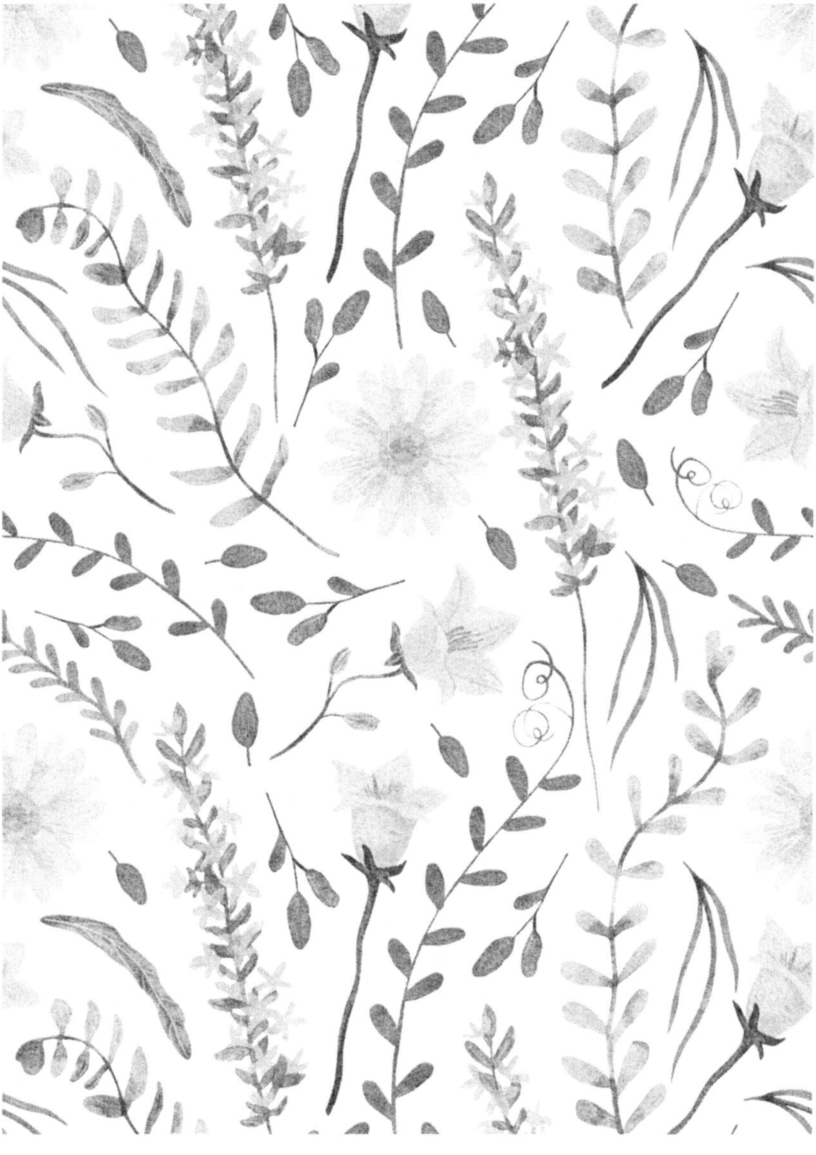

Chapter 4

EVERYDAY WELLNESS AND FIRST AID

It always starts the same way. Maybe it's a sniffle from the backseat on the school run, a stubbed toe in the garden, or that low, familiar throb behind your temples after a long day. You reach for something — but what if that something wasn't a bottle from the drugstore, but a jar from your kitchen shelf?

One rainy afternoon, my daughter came inside from playing, tears in her eyes and a scraped knee that needed more than just a hug. I grabbed the little tin of calendula salve we'd made together the week before — golden, soothing, and smelling faintly of beeswax and sunshine. In that moment, I realized: this is what it means to be prepared. Not with fear or panic, but with presence. With knowledge. With trust in what grows around us.

This chapter is your everyday wellness kit — built from plants, not pills. Whether you're facing a minor burn, a mild cold, or the stress of an overstimulating day, nature offers gentle but powerful support. You don't need to be an herbalist to begin. You just need a few tools, a bit of curiosity, and the willingness to trust your intuition.

Inside, we'll walk through how to build your natural first aid cabinet, one remedy at a time. You'll learn how to soothe bug bites, calm fevers, ease tummy aches, and more — all using ingredients you can grow, buy in bulk, or even forage. We'll also explore immune-boosting tonics, daily teas to support your body through the seasons, and simple strategies for managing everyday stress and tension.

Most importantly, this chapter is about empowerment. It's about that quiet confidence that comes when you know what to reach for — and why. When you begin to see your home not just as a place to live, but as a sanctuary for healing.

Let's begin building that sanctuary, together.

FIRST AID ESSENTIALS: QUICK HERBAL SOLUTIONS

Every household needs a few go-to remedies for those everyday bumps, bruises, and bee stings. Whether you're tending to a skinned knee or a swollen ankle, these quick, plant-based solutions are easy to make, store, and use when you need them most. Think of this section as your natural medicine cabinet — stocked with time-tested herbal allies that offer real relief, fast.

---

1. Calendula Healing Salve

A soothing balm for cuts, scrapes, and irritated skin.

What It's For:
Calendula is a beloved skin-healing herb that gently reduces inflammation, supports tissue repair, and keeps wounds clean. Perfect for minor cuts, scrapes, chapped hands, and diaper rash.

Ingredients:

- 1 cup dried calendula flowers
- 1 cup olive oil (or your choice of carrier oil)
- ¼ cup beeswax pellets
- Optional: a few drops of lavender essential oil

Instructions:

1. Infuse the calendula flowers in oil using a double boiler or sunny windowsill method for 1-2 weeks.
2. Strain out the flowers and gently heat the infused oil with beeswax until melted.
3. Stir in essential oil if using.
4. Pour into tins or jars and let cool.

How to Use:
Apply a thin layer to clean skin as needed. Safe for all ages.

2. Comfrey Compress for Sprains

Support for healing bones, bruises, and sore joints.

What It's For:
Comfrey has been traditionally used to promote tissue and bone repair — earning it the nickname *"knitbone."* Ideal for sprains, strains, and deep bruises.

Ingredients:

- 1 cup dried comfrey leaf or root
- Hot water
- Clean cloth or gauze

Instructions:

1. Steep comfrey in hot water for 15 minutes to create a strong infusion.
2. Soak a cloth in the warm liquid and wring out.
3. Apply to the affected area and cover with a towel. Leave on for 20-30 minutes.

How to Use:

Use 1-2 times daily as needed. Avoid on deep wounds or broken skin.

3. Plantain Poultice for Bug Bites

Nature's antihistamine, right under your feet.

What It's For:
Plantain leaves are a classic remedy for bug bites, bee stings, and splinters. They draw out irritants, reduce itching, and soothe inflammation.

Instructions:

1. Pick a fresh plantain leaf (Plantago major or lanceolata).
2. Chew it briefly or crush with a mortar and pestle to release the juices.
3. Apply directly to the affected area and cover with a bandage. Replace every few hours.

How to Use:

Apply as soon as possible after a sting or bite for best results.

4. Yarrow Powder for Bleeding Wounds

Stop bleeding fast with this battlefield herb.

What It's For:
Yarrow is known for its astringent and antimicrobial properties, making it ideal for stopping minor bleeding and promoting clotting.

Ingredients:
- Dried yarrow leaves and flowers
- Coffee grinder or blender to powder

Instructions:
1. Grind dried yarrow into a fine powder. Store in a clean, dry jar.

How to Use:

Sprinkle directly onto a clean minor cut to slow bleeding. Apply gentle pressure and bandage if needed.

5. Lavender Essential Oil Roll-On for Burns

Instant calm for minor kitchen burns or sunburn.

What It's For:
Lavender essential oil is soothing, antimicrobial, and cooling — ideal for minor burns and skin irritation.

Ingredients:
- 10 ml roller bottle
- 10 drops lavender essential oil
- Carrier oil (like fractionated coconut or jojoba)

Instructions:
1. Fill the roller bottle with carrier oil and essential oil. Shake gently to mix.

How to Use:

Roll gently over the affected area 2-3 times daily. Not for use on open wounds or large burns.

6. Arnica Balm for Bruises

Soothes swelling, bumps, and bruises — naturally.

What It's For:
Arnica is renowned for easing pain, reducing swelling, and speeding up bruise healing. Ideal for minor injuries, sore muscles, and post-workout recovery.

Ingredients:

- 1 cup arnica-infused oil (made with dried arnica flowers + olive oil)
- ¼ cup beeswax pellets
- Optional: 5 drops peppermint or eucalyptus essential oil

Instructions:

1. Gently warm the arnica oil and beeswax together until fully melted.
2. Stir in essential oil if using.
3. Pour into tins and allow to set.

How to Use:

Massage gently into bruised or sore areas 2-3 times daily.

7. Witch Hazel Astringent for Cuts

Nature's toner for wounds and skin care.

What It's For:
Witch hazel is a gentle, effective astringent that helps tighten tissue, reduce bleeding, and cleanse minor cuts or scrapes.

Ingredients:

- ½ cup witch hazel extract (alcohol-based or distilled)
- Optional: 5 drops tea tree or lavender essential oil

Instructions:

1. Combine ingredients in a small glass spray or dropper bottle.

How to Use:

Apply with a clean cotton ball or spray directly on minor wounds. Use before applying a salve or bandage.

8. Aloe Vera Gel for Minor Burns and Skin Irritation

Cooling, hydrating, and skin-soothing.

What It's For:
Aloe vera is a classic remedy for sunburns, small kitchen burns, rashes, and dry or inflamed skin. It cools on contact and promotes gentle healing.

Ingredients:
- 1 fresh aloe vera leaf (or store-bought pure aloe vera gel)
- Optional: a few drops of vitamin E or lavender essential oil

Instructions:
1. Slice open the aloe leaf and scoop out the gel.
2. Blend until smooth for a lotion-like texture.
3. Add optional ingredients and store in the fridge.

How to Use:

Apply directly to irritated or burned skin 2-3 times daily.

---

9. Chamomile Eye Wash

Gentle herbal support for tired, itchy, or irritated eyes.

What It's For:
Chamomile's anti-inflammatory and soothing properties make it ideal for eye strain, seasonal allergies, or minor eye irritation.

Ingredients:
- 1 tsp dried chamomile flowers
- 1 cup boiled, distilled water

Instructions:
1. Steep chamomile in freshly boiled water for 10-15 minutes.
2. Strain thoroughly through a fine cloth or filter. Let cool completely.
3. Use with a sterile eye cup or clean cotton pad.

How to Use:

Gently rinse eyes or apply as a compress. Use only once per batch; discard leftovers.

Always strain very well — no herbal bits should remain.

10. Goldenseal Root Antiseptic Wash

Potent antimicrobial for cleansing wounds and infections.

What It's For:
Goldenseal has strong antibacterial properties and has long been used to cleanse wounds and prevent infection.

Ingredients:

- 1 tsp dried goldenseal root
- 1 cup boiled distilled water

Instructions:

1. Simmer goldenseal in water for 10 minutes.
2. Strain well and let cool.
3. Store in a clean, sterilized jar and use within 24 hours.

How to Use:

Use as a wash for minor cuts, abrasions, or skin infections. Dab with clean cloth or gauze.

EVERYDAY WELLNESS: BOOSTING IMMUNITY NATURALLY

A strong immune system doesn't come from one magic pill — it's gently nurtured, season by season. Whether it's cold and flu season or just a hectic week, your body needs support to stay balanced and resilient. The good news? Nature offers powerful allies. This section includes everyday tonics, broths, and tinctures to help fortify your defenses, gently and consistently. These are simple remedies you can make in your own kitchen — no lab coat required.

11. Elderberry Syrup

A delicious immune booster for cold and flu season.

What It's For:
Rich in antioxidants and antiviral properties, elderberries are a go-to for reducing the duration and severity of colds and flu.

Ingredients:

- 1 cup dried elderberries
- 3 cups water

- 1 cinnamon stick
- 4-5 whole cloves
- 1-inch piece fresh ginger, sliced
- ¾ cup raw honey (or maple syrup for vegan option)

Instructions:

1. Combine elderberries, water, cinnamon, cloves, and ginger in a saucepan.
2. Bring to a boil, then simmer uncovered for 30-40 minutes, until reduced by half.
3. Cool slightly, then strain into a bowl.
4. Stir in honey and store in a glass jar in the fridge.

How to Use:

Take 1 tablespoon daily for prevention, or every 2-3 hours if symptoms arise.

For kids over 1 year: 1 teaspoon.

---

12. Astragalus Immunity Broth

A nourishing base for soups and stews that supports long-term vitality.

What It's For:

Astragalus root is a deeply restorative adaptogen that supports immune health over time. Great for the whole family.

Ingredients:

- 3-5 slices dried astragalus root
- 1 onion, chopped
- 2 carrots, chopped
- 2 celery stalks, chopped
- 3 cloves garlic
- 8 cups water
- Optional: fresh herbs (parsley, thyme), seaweed, or mushrooms

Instructions:

1. Combine all ingredients in a large pot and bring to a boil.
2. Simmer for 1-2 hours.
3. Strain and use as a base for soups, or sip as a nourishing tea.

How to Use:

Drink 1-2 cups several times a week during cold seasons. Freeze extra broth in jars or cubes.

13. Olive Leaf Extract Tonic

Potent antimicrobial support from a Mediterranean classic.

What It's For:

Olive leaf is known for its antiviral and antibacterial properties — helpful during colds, flu, or as a preventive tonic.

Ingredients:

- 1 tbsp dried olive leaves (or 30 drops olive leaf tincture)
- 1 cup water
- Optional: honey and lemon for flavor

Instructions:

1. Simmer dried olive leaf in water for 10-15 minutes.
2. Strain and drink as tea, or add tincture to warm water.
3. Sweeten to taste.

How to Use:

Drink 1 cup daily during cold season or at first sign of illness.

14. Echinacea-Ginger Tincture

A bold boost when you feel a cold coming on.

What It's For:

Echinacea is known for stimulating immune activity, especially at the onset of illness. Ginger adds warmth and circulatory support.

Ingredients:

- ½ cup dried echinacea root
- 2 tablespoons fresh ginger, chopped
- 1 cup 80-100 proof vodka or brandy
- Glass jar with lid

Instructions:

1. Place herbs in a jar and cover with alcohol.
2. Seal, shake gently, and store in a cool, dark place for 3-4 weeks.
3. Strain into a dropper bottle.

How to Use:

At first sign of illness, take 1 dropperful (about 30 drops) every 2-3 hours. Best used short-term, not daily for prevention.

15. Garlic-Honey Oxymel

A sweet and tangy immune tonic with serious punch.

What It's For:
Garlic is a natural antimicrobial powerhouse, and when combined with raw honey and apple cider vinegar, it becomes a tasty, immune-loving elixir.

Ingredients:
- 1 head fresh garlic, peeled and crushed
- ½ cup raw apple cider vinegar
- ½ cup raw honey

Instructions:
1. Mix crushed garlic with vinegar and honey in a glass jar.
2. Shake well and let sit for 1-2 weeks, shaking daily.
3. Strain (optional) and store in the fridge.

How to Use:

Take 1 teaspoon daily as prevention, or every few hours when sick.

Can also drizzle on salads or mix into warm water.

16. Reishi Mushroom Elixir

Calming, nourishing, and deeply immune-supportive.

What It's For:
Reishi is an adaptogen that supports immune regulation, stress relief, and restful sleep. Best used consistently over time.

Ingredients:
- ½ cup dried reishi mushroom slices
- 4 cups water
- Optional: cinnamon stick, vanilla, or cacao powder for flavor

Instructions:
1. Simmer reishi and any optional spices in water for 30-60 minutes.
2. Strain and sip warm.
3. Sweeten lightly with honey if desired.

How to Use:

Drink ½ to 1 cup daily, especially during high-stress or low-energy periods.

17. Turmeric-Ginger Shots

A daily anti-inflammatory kick to support immunity and vitality.

What It's For:
Turmeric and ginger are both powerful anti-inflammatory and immune-supportive roots. These vibrant wellness shots are great for daily prevention and reducing inflammation.

Ingredients:
- ¼ cup fresh turmeric root, chopped (or 2 tsp ground)
- ¼ cup fresh ginger root, chopped
- Juice of 2 lemons
- 1-2 tablespoons raw honey
- 1 cup water
- Pinch of black pepper (enhances turmeric absorption)

Instructions:
1. Blend all ingredients until smooth.
2. Strain through cheesecloth or a fine strainer.
3. Pour into a glass jar or small shot bottles and refrigerate.

How to Use:

Take 1-2 ounces daily. Shake well before using.

Use caution with turmeric if pregnant or on blood thinners.

---

18. Mushroom-Infused Bone Broth

Deep nourishment for immunity, gut health, and strength.

What It's For:
This mineral-rich broth combines the immune-boosting powers of mushrooms with the gut-healing properties of traditional bone broth.

Ingredients:
- 1 lb bones (chicken, beef, or veggie-based if preferred)
- ½ cup mixed dried medicinal mushrooms (shiitake, reishi, maitake, etc.)
- 1 onion, 2 carrots, 2 celery stalks
- 3 cloves garlic
- 1 tbsp apple cider vinegar
- 10 cups water

Instructions:

1. Combine all ingredients in a large pot or slow cooker.
2. Simmer for 12-24 hours.
3. Strain and store in the fridge or freezer.

How to Use:

Sip 1 cup daily or use as a base for soups, grains, or savory herbal tonics.

---

19. Vitamin C Herbal Infusion (Rosehips + Hibiscus)

A tangy, antioxidant-rich tea for daily wellness.

What It's For:

Rosehips and hibiscus are both rich in vitamin C and antioxidants, supporting immune health and healthy skin.

Ingredients:

- 1 tbsp dried rosehips
- 1 tbsp dried hibiscus flowers
- 2 cups boiled water
- Optional: orange peel or cinnamon stick

Instructions:

1. Steep herbs in hot water for 20-30 minutes, covered.
2. Strain and enjoy warm or chilled.
3. Add honey or a splash of juice if desired.

How to Use:

Drink 1-2 cups daily. Beautiful served iced in summer!

---

20. Fire Cider (Spicy Immunity Tonic)

A zesty, warming infusion for cold days and sluggish systems.

What It's For:

Fire cider stimulates circulation, digestion, and immune response. This folk remedy is a spicy, vinegar-based infusion loaded with warming herbs and roots.

Ingredients:

- ½ cup grated horseradish
- ½ cup chopped onion

- ¼ cup minced garlic
- ¼ cup grated ginger
- 1 sliced jalapeño (optional)
- 1 lemon, sliced
- Raw apple cider vinegar (enough to cover)
- Raw honey, to taste (added after straining)

Instructions:

1. Add all ingredients (except honey) to a large jar.
2. Cover with vinegar, seal, and shake well.
3. Steep for 3-4 weeks in a cool, dark place. Shake daily.
4. Strain and mix in honey to taste.

How to Use:

Take 1 tablespoon daily, or more frequently when sick.

Also great as a salad dressing or marinade!

HERBAL TEAS FOR COMMON AILMENTS

There's something profoundly soothing about wrapping your hands around a warm mug of herbal tea. It's more than just a drink — it's a ritual, a remedy, and a moment of pause. In this section, we'll explore simple herbal infusions designed to support common discomforts: digestion, stress, colds, and more. Each blend is easy to prepare, gentle enough for daily use, and deeply rooted in traditional wisdom. Whether you're steeping a single herb or combining a few, these teas offer real support — and a little bit of comfort — exactly when you need it most.

---

21. Lemon Balm Tea

A gentle mood lifter for anxious or cloudy days.

What It's For:

Lemon balm is a nervine — it calms the mind, lifts the spirits, and supports restful sleep. Ideal for stress, mild anxiety, or emotional overwhelm.

Ingredients:

- 1-2 tsp dried lemon balm leaves
- 1 cup boiling water

Instructions:

1. Steep lemon balm in hot water for 10-15 minutes.
2. Strain and sip slowly.

How to Use:

Enjoy up to 2-3 cups daily as needed. Also lovely before bed.

---

22. Fennel Seed Tea

Soothes bloating, gas, and sluggish digestion.

What It's For:

Fennel seeds relax the digestive tract, reduce gas, and stimulate gentle detoxification. Great after heavy meals or when dealing with bloating.

Ingredients:

- 1 tsp crushed fennel seeds
- 1 cup boiling water

Instructions:

1. Crush seeds lightly in a mortar and pestle.
2. Steep in hot water for 10-15 minutes. Strain.

How to Use:

Drink after meals or anytime you feel bloated or uncomfortable.

Safe during breastfeeding — can also help ease colic in infants via mom's milk.

---

23. Ginger & Licorice Root Tea

A sweet, warming brew for colds, coughs, and sore throats.

What It's For:

Ginger warms the body and supports circulation, while licorice soothes sore throats and supports adrenal balance. A beautiful ally for early colds or winter blues.

Ingredients:

- 1 tbsp fresh ginger, sliced (or 1 tsp dried)
- 1 tsp dried licorice root
- 2 cups water

Instructions:

1. Simmer herbs gently in water for 10-15 minutes.
2. Strain and sweeten with honey if desired.

How to Use:

Drink 1-2 cups as needed.

Avoid licorice if you have high blood pressure or are pregnant.

---

24. Hibiscus Tea

A tart, cooling tea that supports heart health and healthy blood pressure.

What It's For:

Hibiscus is high in antioxidants and shown to help regulate blood pressure. It's also deeply refreshing and supportive of the cardiovascular system.

Ingredients:

- 1 tbsp dried hibiscus petals
- 2 cups boiling water

Instructions:

1. Steep petals for 15-20 minutes.
2. Strain and sweeten if desired with honey or fruit juice.

How to Use:

Drink 1-2 cups daily. Delicious hot or iced.

Avoid in pregnancy due to its potential to affect hormone balance.

---

25. Cinnamon & Clove Tea

A warming digestive tea that helps balance blood sugar.

What It's For:

Cinnamon and clove both support healthy blood sugar levels and curb sweet cravings, while also warming the body and aiding digestion.

Ingredients:

- 1 cinnamon stick (or 1 tsp ground)
- 2-3 whole cloves
- 1½ cups boiling water

Instructions:

1. Simmer spices gently in water for 10-15 minutes.
2. Strain and enjoy warm, optionally with a splash of milk or honey.

How to Use:

Drink once or twice daily after meals.

Cinnamon is stimulating in high doses — enjoy in moderation.

---

26. Mullein Leaf Tea

A gentle lung tonic to support clear breathing and respiratory health.

What It's For:

Mullein soothes the respiratory tract, supports lung function, and helps clear congestion. Excellent during coughs, colds, or allergy season.

Ingredients:

- 1 tbsp dried mullein leaf
- 1½ cups boiling water

Instructions:

1. Steep mullein in hot water for 15 minutes.
2. Strain **very well** through a fine filter or cloth to remove tiny hairs.

How to Use:

Drink 1-3 cups daily during respiratory challenges or recovery.

Great as a steam or gargle, too!

---

27. Chamomile & Peppermint Tea

A calming blend for upset stomachs and digestive ease.

What It's For:

Chamomile soothes the gut and calms the nervous system, while peppermint eases cramping, gas, and bloating. Perfect after meals or when tension settles in the belly.

Ingredients:

- 1 tsp dried chamomile flowers
- 1 tsp dried peppermint leaves
- 1½ cups boiling water

Instructions:

1. Combine herbs in a mug or teapot.
2. Pour boiling water over them.
3. Cover and steep for 10-15 minutes. Strain and sip warm.

How to Use:

Drink after meals or at bedtime. Safe for children in small amounts.

---

28. Nettle & Raspberry Leaf Tea

Gentle support for energy, minerals, and iron — especially for women.

What It's For:

Nettle is rich in iron and minerals, while raspberry leaf tones the uterus and supports hormonal balance. A favorite for menstruating, pregnant, or postpartum bodies.

Ingredients:

- 1 tbsp dried nettle leaf
- 1 tbsp dried raspberry leaf
- 2 cups boiling water

Instructions:

1. Steep herbs in a covered jar or teapot for 15-30 minutes.
2. Strain and enjoy warm or iced.

How to Use:

Drink daily as a mineral-rich tonic.

Avoid raspberry leaf in early pregnancy unless advised.

---

29. Linden & Elderflower Tea

A gentle sweat-inducing tea to support fevers and colds.

What It's For:

Both linden and elderflower are classic diaphoretics — they encourage gentle sweating to help the body manage fever. This blend also calms nerves and supports rest.

Ingredients:

- 1 tsp dried linden flowers
- 1 tsp dried elderflowers

- 1½ cups boiling water

Instructions:

1. Steep herbs in hot water for 10-15 minutes.
2. Strain and sip warm, bundled up to promote sweating.

How to Use:

Drink 2-3 cups per day during colds, fevers, or chills. Especially helpful at the onset of illness.

---

30. Valerian Root & Skullcap Tea

A strong, sedating blend for deep sleep and nervous tension.

What It's For:

Valerian root is a natural sedative that promotes restful sleep, while skullcap soothes frazzled nerves and tension. Ideal for occasional insomnia or overactive minds.

Ingredients:

- ½ tsp dried valerian root
- 1 tsp dried skullcap
- 1½ cups boiling water

Instructions:

1. Steep herbs for 10-15 minutes, covered.
2. Strain and drink 30-60 minutes before bed.

How to Use:

Use occasionally as needed for sleep support.

Valerian may cause vivid dreams or grogginess in some people — start with a small amount.

TINCTURES AND TONICS FOR ENERGY AND VITALITY

Energy isn't just about staying awake — it's about feeling vibrant, focused, and resilient in your daily life. Whether you're recovering from burnout, juggling too many roles, or simply looking for natural support to stay steady and strong, adaptogenic herbs and energizing tonics can help restore balance. This section focuses on tinctures and tonics designed to nourish the nervous system, balance stress hormones, and support sustainable energy — without the crash. These blends are simple to make and powerful when used consistently, helping you feel more grounded, clear-headed, and capable — one drop at a time.

---

31. Ginseng & Schisandra Tincture

A revitalizing blend for focus, stamina, and endurance.

What It's For:
Ginseng supports physical and mental energy, while schisandra berries enhance clarity, endurance, and liver function. Together, they form a powerful tonic for active or high-stress lifestyles.

Ingredients:

- 2 tbsp dried American or Asian ginseng root
- 1 tbsp dried schisandra berries
- 1 cup 80-100 proof vodka or brandy
- Glass jar with lid

Instructions:

1. Combine herbs in a jar and cover with alcohol.
2. Seal, shake, and store in a cool, dark place for 3-4 weeks.
3. Strain and bottle.

How to Use:

Take 1-2 dropperfuls in the morning or early afternoon.

Avoid late-day use, especially for sensitive sleepers.

---

32. Maca Energy Blend

A grounding, hormone-balancing powder for sustained energy.

What It's For:
Maca root is a traditional Andean adaptogen that supports stamina, libido, and hormone balance — especially helpful during hormonal shifts or fatigue.

Ingredients:

- 2 tbsp maca root powder
- 1 tbsp cacao powder
- ½ tsp cinnamon
- Optional: pinch of cayenne

Instructions:

1. Mix ingredients and store in a sealed jar.

How to Use:

Add 1 tsp to smoothies, coffee, warm milk, or oatmeal. Use daily or as needed.

---

33. Rhodiola Adaptogenic Tonic

Builds resilience to stress and sharpens mental clarity.

What It's For:

Rhodiola rosea is a beloved adaptogen for enhancing mental performance, physical stamina, and emotional resilience, especially under pressure.

Ingredients:

- 1 tbsp dried rhodiola root
- 1 cup 80-100 proof vodka or brandy

Instructions:

1. Place rhodiola in a jar and cover with alcohol.
2. Steep for 3-4 weeks, shaking occasionally.
3. Strain and store in a dropper bottle.

How to Use:

Take ½ to 1 dropperful in the morning or before mentally demanding tasks. Best for short-term or cyclic use, not daily long-term.

---

34. Ashwagandha Stress-Resilience Tincture

A gentle, grounding adaptogen for restoring calm and steady energy.

What It's For:

Ashwagandha helps rebuild the body's stress tolerance, supports sleep, and balances adrenal health. Ideal for burnout, anxiety, or chronic fatigue.

Ingredients:

- 2 tbsp dried ashwagandha root
- 1 cup vodka, brandy, or apple cider vinegar (for alcohol-free)
- Glass jar with lid

Instructions:

1. Combine ingredients and steep for 3-4 weeks.
2. Strain and store in a dark glass bottle.

How to Use:

Take 1 dropperful once or twice daily.

Especially effective taken consistently for several weeks.

---

35. Green Tea & Gotu Kola Tonic

Gentle stimulation for mental clarity, focus, and creative energy.

What It's For:
Green tea provides clean caffeine and antioxidant power, while gotu kola nourishes brain function and circulation without overstimulation.

Ingredients:

- 1 tsp loose-leaf green tea
- 1 tsp dried gotu kola
- 2 cups hot (not boiling) water

Instructions:

1. Steep herbs for 5-10 minutes in hot water (not boiling, to preserve green tea benefits).
2. Strain and enjoy warm or iced.

How to Use:

Drink in the morning or early afternoon to support clear, focused energy.

Can add a splash of lemon or mint for freshness.

---

36. Holy Basil (Tulsi) Morning Elixir

A heart-opening adaptogen for calm clarity and emotional energy.

What It's For:
Tulsi is a beloved Ayurvedic herb that lifts the mood, balances stress hormones, and gently energizes without overstimulation — perfect for starting your day grounded and focused.

Ingredients:

- 1 tsp dried tulsi leaves (or 1 tbsp fresh)
- Juice of ½ lemon
- 1 tsp raw honey
- 1½ cups hot water (not boiling)

Instructions:

1. Steep tulsi leaves in hot water for 10-15 minutes.
2. Strain, then stir in lemon juice and honey.
3. Sip mindfully in the morning.

How to Use:

Enjoy daily as part of your morning ritual or during emotional stress.

---

37. Bee Pollen & Honey Shot

A nutrient-rich boost to start the day with natural vitality.

What It's For:

Bee pollen is packed with B vitamins, protein, and antioxidants, supporting energy and immune health. Combined with honey, it becomes a simple, delicious power-up.

Ingredients:

- 1 tsp bee pollen granules
- 1 tsp raw honey
- Optional: splash of lemon juice or sprinkle of cinnamon

Instructions:

1. Mix bee pollen and honey into a small spoonful or shot glass.
2. Stir in optional additions.

How to Use:

Take first thing in the morning or before exercise.

Not suitable for those with pollen allergies.

---

38. Cordyceps Mushroom Tonic

A powerhouse tonic for stamina, endurance, and oxygen flow.

What It's For:

Cordyceps mushrooms are renowned for boosting physical energy, lung capacity, and endurance — often used by athletes and those recovering from fatigue.

Ingredients:

- 1 tbsp dried cordyceps
- 2 cups water
- Optional: cinnamon or cacao for flavor

Instructions:

1. Simmer cordyceps in water for 30 minutes.
2. Strain and enjoy warm or chilled.
3. Add optional ingredients to taste.

How to Use:

Drink ½-1 cup before workouts or during energy slumps.

---

39. Suma Root Energy Blend

Also known as "Brazilian ginseng," suma is a strength and vitality tonic.

What It's For:

Suma root supports hormone balance, energy, and recovery — particularly useful for athletes, menstruating individuals, and those under chronic stress.

Ingredients:

- 1 tbsp suma root powder
- 1 tbsp maca powder
- 1 tsp cacao powder
- Warm nut milk or smoothie base

Instructions:

1. Blend powders into warm milk or smoothie.
2. Sweeten with honey or maple syrup if desired.

How to Use:

Drink daily or before physical activity.

Avoid during pregnancy or with hormone-sensitive conditions.

---

40. Siberian Ginseng Tea Tonic

A balancing brew for long-term stamina and immune strength.

What It's For:

Siberian ginseng (Eleuthero) is a gentle adaptogen that boosts resilience, supports adrenal function, and enhances endurance without being overstimulating.

Ingredients:

- 1 tbsp dried Siberian ginseng root
- 2 cups water

Instructions:

1. Simmer root in water for 20-30 minutes.
2. Strain and enjoy plain or with lemon and honey.

How to Use:

Drink 1 cup in the morning, several times a week for ongoing support.
Best taken in cycles (3-4 weeks on, 1 week off).

STRESS AND ANXIETY RELIEF WITH HERBAL REMEDIES

Stress is part of life — but so is restoration. When the world feels too loud or your to-do list too long, herbs can offer a quiet, steady kind of support. This section includes simple, heart-soothing remedies to ease anxiety, encourage restful sleep, and bring the nervous system back into balance. Whether it's a calming tea, a relaxing bath, or a tincture you tuck into your bag, these gentle allies are here to remind you: you are safe, and healing can be soft.

---

41. Lavender & Chamomile Oil Blend

A calming massage or diffuser oil to ease tension and restlessness.

What It's For:

Both lavender and chamomile are beloved for their soothing effects on the nervous system. This blend supports deep relaxation, especially at bedtime or during anxious moments.

Ingredients:

- 10 drops lavender essential oil
- 5 drops Roman chamomile essential oil
- 2 tbsp carrier oil (like sweet almond or jojoba)

Instructions:

1. Combine oils in a glass bottle.
2. Shake gently to blend.

How to Use:

Massage onto neck, chest, or feet before bed, or use in a diffuser.
Safe for kids in lower dilution (2-3 drops total).

42. Passionflower Tincture

A gentle sedative herb for racing thoughts and nighttime anxiety.

What It's For:
Passionflower supports calm by quieting circular thoughts and promoting restful sleep. Ideal for bedtime or moments of overwhelm.

Ingredients:

- 2 tbsp dried passionflower
- 1 cup vodka or brandy
- Glass jar with lid

Instructions:

1. Combine herb and alcohol in a jar.
2. Steep for 4 weeks, shaking gently every few days.
3. Strain and bottle.

How to Use:

Take 1-2 dropperfuls in the evening or as needed for anxiety.

Avoid combining with sedative medications.

43. Lemon Balm Sleep Spray

An aromatic mist to signal your body that it's time to rest.

What It's For:
Lemon balm helps ease anxiety and calm the mind, while lavender encourages rest. This pillow spray is a simple ritual to wind down the day.

Ingredients:

- ½ cup distilled water
- 1 tbsp lemon balm tincture or hydrosol
- 5 drops lavender essential oil
- 1 tsp witch hazel (helps oils disperse)

Instructions:

1. Combine all ingredients in a 2 oz spray bottle.
2. Shake before each use.

How to Use:

Spritz onto your pillow, bedding, or into the air before bedtime.

44. Holy Basil Tea for Calm

A daily ritual for emotional balance and stress resilience.

What It's For:
Holy basil (tulsi) helps regulate cortisol and soothe the heart. It's an ideal everyday tea for managing chronic stress and emotional fatigue.

Ingredients:
- 1-2 tsp dried tulsi leaves
- 1½ cups hot (not boiling) water

Instructions:
1. Steep leaves for 10-15 minutes.
2. Strain and sip slowly, ideally in a quiet space.

How to Use:
Drink 1-3 cups daily for ongoing nervous system support.

---

45. Adaptogenic Stress Gummies

A fun and functional way to support stress resilience daily.

What It's For:
These gummies combine calming adaptogens like ashwagandha or tulsi with a tasty base — perfect for on-the-go stress support or as part of a calming ritual.

Ingredients:
- 1 cup strong herbal tea (e.g., tulsi, ashwagandha, or lemon balm)
- 1 tbsp grass-fed gelatin (or vegan alternative like agar agar)
- 1-2 tbsp honey or maple syrup
- Silicone gummy molds

Instructions:
1. Heat herbal tea until warm (not boiling), then whisk in gelatin until dissolved.
2. Stir in sweetener.
3. Pour into molds and chill for 1-2 hours.
4. Pop out and store in the fridge for up to a week.

How to Use:
Enjoy 1-2 gummies as a daily stress support or calming treat.

46. Valerian Sleep Drops

A quick, effective support for sleepless nights or restless minds.

What It's For:
Valerian root helps ease tension and promote deeper, uninterrupted sleep. This tincture is fast-acting and perfect when winding down feels impossible.

Ingredients:
- 2 tbsp dried valerian root
- 1 cup vodka or brandy
- Amber glass dropper bottle

Instructions:
1. Combine valerian and alcohol in a jar and steep for 3-4 weeks.
2. Shake every few days.
3. Strain and bottle.

How to Use:

Take 1 dropperful 30-60 minutes before bed.

Start small — valerian can be very potent.

47. Stress Relief Inhaler (Essential Oil Blend)

A discreet, quick-acting blend to calm the mind anytime, anywhere.

What It's For:
Aromatic compounds from essential oils reach the brain quickly via the olfactory system, helping to calm anxiety, clear overwhelm, and promote presence.

Ingredients:
- 5 drops lavender essential oil
- 4 drops bergamot
- 3 drops frankincense
- 2 drops Roman chamomile
- 1 blank inhaler (cotton wick + case)

Instructions:
1. Add essential oils to the cotton wick.
2. Insert into inhaler and seal tightly.

How to Use:

Inhale deeply through each nostril as needed during stressful moments.

48. Kava Root Chill Tonic

A deeply relaxing tonic for winding down without drowsiness.

What It's For:
Kava is a traditional South Pacific herb known for relaxing the muscles, calming the mind, and enhancing sociability. It's perfect for stress relief without sedation.

Ingredients:
- 1 tbsp powdered kava root
- 1 cup cool water or plant milk
- Optional: cinnamon, vanilla, or cocoa

Instructions:
1. Place kava in a muslin bag or cloth.
2. Knead and squeeze in cool liquid for 5-10 minutes.
3. Strain and flavor as desired.

How to Use:

Drink in the evening or socially to unwind.

Avoid with alcohol or liver issues. Use occasionally, not daily.

49. Magnesium & Lavender Bath Soak

A relaxing mineral-rich soak to ease muscle tension and mental stress.

What It's For:
Magnesium helps relax muscles and supports the nervous system. Lavender soothes the senses and prepares the body for sleep.

Ingredients:
- 1 cup Epsom salts
- ½ cup baking soda
- 10 drops lavender essential oil
- Optional: ¼ cup dried lavender or chamomile flowers

Instructions:
1. Mix all ingredients and store in a jar.
2. Add ½-1 cup to warm bath water and soak for 20-30 minutes.

How to Use:

Use before bed or anytime you need deep, physical relaxation.

50. Aromatherapy Pillow Spray

A dreamy blend to turn your bedroom into a calming sanctuary.

What It's For:
This spray helps ease nighttime tension and prepares the senses for rest. Lavender, cedarwood, and sweet orange create a soft, grounding aroma.

Ingredients:

- ½ cup distilled water
- 1 tsp witch hazel or vodka
- 5 drops lavender essential oil
- 3 drops cedarwood
- 2 drops sweet orange
- Small spray bottle

Instructions:

1. Combine all ingredients in the bottle.
2. Shake well before each use.

How to Use:

Spritz onto pillows, sheets, or into the air 5-10 minutes before bedtime.

NATURAL SOLUTIONS FOR COLD AND FLU

When cold and flu season strikes, having simple, natural remedies on hand can make all the difference. From stubborn coughs to stuffy noses, these herbal supports help ease symptoms, boost recovery, and bring comfort to the whole family — without reaching for harsh medications. This section includes warming syrups, soothing steams, and immune-loving teas that are easy to make and safe to share. Whether you're caring for yourself or a loved one, these remedies remind us: healing often begins with warmth, rest, and a little help from the herbs.

51. Elderberry-Ginger Lozenges

Immune-boosting and throat-soothing treats for cold season.

What It's For:
Elderberries are antiviral, and ginger helps reduce inflammation and fight infection — perfect for sore throats or early symptoms.

Ingredients:

- ½ cup elderberry syrup (see Recipe 11)
- 2 tsp powdered ginger
- 2 tbsp lemon juice
- 2 cups sugar (or coconut sugar)
- Candy thermometer, silicone mold or parchment paper

Instructions:

1. Combine ingredients in a saucepan and bring to a boil.
2. Simmer until it reaches 300°F (hard crack stage).
3. Pour into molds or drop onto parchment. Let cool and harden.
4. Dust with arrowroot to prevent sticking.

How to Use:

Suck on 1 lozenge as needed for sore throat or immune support.

---

52. Herbal Chest Rub (Thyme, Eucalyptus, Peppermint)

A DIY vapor rub to ease cough, open airways, and relax tight breathing.

What It's For:

Thyme is antimicrobial, eucalyptus clears the lungs, and peppermint cools and relieves tightness. This balm is a natural alternative to store-bought menthol rubs.

Ingredients:

- ½ cup coconut oil or shea butter
- ¼ cup beeswax pellets
- 10 drops eucalyptus essential oil
- 8 drops peppermint essential oil
- 5 drops thyme essential oil

Instructions:

1. Gently melt coconut oil and beeswax in a double boiler.
2. Remove from heat and stir in essential oils.
3. Pour into tins and allow to set.

How to Use:

Rub on chest, upper back, and bottoms of feet during congestion or coughs. Avoid applying to the face or using on infants.

53. Steam Inhalation with Eucalyptus & Thyme

Opens sinuses and soothes congestion with herbal vapors.

What It's For:
Steam inhalation helps break up mucus and ease breathing. Eucalyptus opens airways, and thyme offers antibacterial support.

Ingredients:

- 1 tbsp dried thyme
- 3-4 drops eucalyptus essential oil
- Large bowl of hot water
- Towel

Instructions:

1. Place thyme in the bowl and pour in boiling water.
2. Add essential oil.
3. Drape a towel over your head and inhale the steam for 5-10 minutes.

How to Use:

Use 1-2 times daily during congestion or sinus pressure.

Not recommended for very young children due to strong oils.

54. Onion & Honey Cough Syrup

A classic folk remedy that breaks up mucus and calms the cough.

What It's For:
Raw onion has natural expectorant properties, while honey soothes irritated throats and calms the cough reflex.

Ingredients:

- 1 small organic onion, thinly sliced
- ½ cup raw honey

Instructions:

1. Layer onion slices and honey in a clean jar.
2. Let sit for 8-12 hours at room temperature.
3. Strain out the onion and keep the syrup in the fridge.

How to Use:

Take 1 tsp every 2-3 hours for cough or congestion.

Do not give honey to children under 1 year old.

55. Throat-Soothing Sage Tea

An herbal tea or gargle for sore, inflamed throats.

What It's For:
Sage has astringent, antibacterial, and anti-inflammatory properties — perfect for sore throats, swollen tonsils, or dry coughs.

Ingredients:
- 1 tsp dried sage leaf
- 1 cup boiling water
- Optional: lemon juice, honey

Instructions:
1. Steep sage in boiling water for 10 minutes.
2. Strain and sip slowly, or cool and use as a gargle.

How to Use:

Drink 1-3 times daily or gargle every few hours for throat relief.

Avoid large internal doses during pregnancy.

56. Garlic Oil Ear Drops

A traditional remedy for earaches and infections.

What It's For:
Garlic is naturally antimicrobial and anti-inflammatory. Infused in oil, it provides gentle relief for mild ear discomfort or early infections.

Ingredients:
- 2-3 cloves fresh garlic, chopped
- ¼ cup olive oil
- Small dropper bottle

Instructions:
1. Gently warm garlic in olive oil over low heat for 10-15 minutes. Do not let it sizzle.
2. Cool completely and strain. Store in the fridge.

How to Use:

Warm slightly, then place 1-2 drops in the affected ear (not if eardrum is perforated).

Always check with a healthcare provider if symptoms persist.

57. Sinus-Clearing Herbal Nasal Spray

A gentle, natural spray to reduce sinus pressure and open nasal passages.

What It's For:

Salt water relieves congestion, while herbs like goldenseal and thyme provide antimicrobial support. This spray helps clear blocked sinuses and reduce infection risk.

Ingredients:

- 1 cup distilled or boiled, cooled water
- ¼ tsp sea salt
- ¼ tsp baking soda
- Optional: 10 drops thyme or goldenseal tincture
- Clean nasal spray bottle

Instructions:

1. Mix ingredients and pour into a clean spray bottle.
2. Shake gently before use.

How to Use:

Spray 1-2 times in each nostril up to 3x daily.

Discard and refresh every 3-5 days. Not for infants.

58. Licorice Root Cough Tea

A naturally sweet tea that soothes the throat and calms coughing fits.

What It's For:

Licorice is a demulcent herb — it coats and soothes irritated mucous membranes while supporting the adrenals and calming inflammation.

Ingredients:

- 1 tsp dried licorice root
- 1 tsp slippery elm bark (optional)
- 1½ cups boiling water

Instructions:

1. Steep herbs for 10-15 minutes, covered.
2. Strain and sip warm.

How to Use:

Drink 1-2 cups daily during cough or throat irritation.

Avoid licorice with high blood pressure or during pregnancy unless supervised.

59. Mullein & Marshmallow Syrup

A gentle, lung-loving syrup for dry coughs and irritated throats.

What It's For:
Mullein opens the lungs and eases coughing, while marshmallow root soothes inflammation and irritation. This combo is perfect for dry, persistent coughs.

Ingredients:
- 1 tbsp dried mullein leaf
- 1 tbsp dried marshmallow root
- 2 cups water
- ½-¾ cup raw honey

Instructions:
1. Simmer herbs in water for 30 minutes.
2. Strain through a fine cloth to remove mullein fuzz.
3. Stir in honey while warm, not hot.
4. Bottle and refrigerate.

How to Use:

Take 1 tsp every 2-3 hours for dry, tickly coughs. Safe for children over 1 year.

60. Immune Bomb Essential Oil Blend

A potent, protective diffuser or topical blend for fighting off infection.

What It's For:
This blend combines antiviral, antibacterial, and immune-stimulating essential oils to help purify the air, support the immune system, and reduce germ exposure.

Ingredients:
- 5 drops tea tree essential oil
- 5 drops eucalyptus
- 4 drops lemon
- 3 drops rosemary
- 3 drops clove
- Optional carrier oil (for topical use)

Instructions:
1. Blend essential oils and store in a dark glass bottle.

2. For diffusion, use 3-5 drops in a diffuser.
3. For topical use, dilute in 2 tbsp carrier oil.

How to Use:

Diffuse during cold season or apply to the chest, feet, or neck (always patch test first).

Not recommended for children under 10 or during pregnancy.

ALLERGY RELIEF: HERBAL SOLUTIONS FOR SEASONAL ALLERGIES

When spring blooms or fall winds kick up sneezes, itchy eyes, and sinus pressure, turning to nature for relief — instead of reacting to it — is a powerful shift. Seasonal allergies are your body's response to irritation, and herbal remedies can help soothe that response without the grogginess or side effects of conventional meds. This section includes gentle, effective supports that help modulate the immune system, reduce inflammation, and calm histamine reactions naturally. With the right herbs and habits, allergy season doesn't have to mean suffering.

---

61. Nettle Leaf Capsules

A natural antihistamine to calm allergy flares from the inside out.

What It's For:

Nettle leaf is rich in nutrients and helps reduce histamine response, easing symptoms like sneezing, itching, and runny nose.

Ingredients:

- Dried nettle leaf powder
- Empty size 00 capsules (and capsule machine or by hand)

Instructions:

1. Fill capsules with nettle powder.
2. Store in a glass jar away from light and moisture.

How to Use:

Take 2 capsules (about 1,000 mg) 1-2 times daily during allergy season.

Can also be used as tea, but capsules are more concentrated.

62. Quercetin Herbal Tincture

Supports immune balance and reduces allergy inflammation.

What It's For:
Quercetin is a plant compound known for stabilizing mast cells (which release histamine). Combined with anti-inflammatory herbs, it becomes a powerful seasonal support.

Ingredients:
- 1 tbsp dried nettle leaf
- 1 tbsp dried ginkgo or eyebright
- 1 tbsp chopped onion peel (natural source of quercetin)
- 1 cup vodka or brandy

Instructions:
1. Place herbs in a jar, cover with alcohol, and steep for 3-4 weeks.
2. Shake every few days, then strain and store in a dropper bottle.

How to Use:

Take 1-2 dropperfuls twice daily during high-allergen times.

Not for use during pregnancy or while taking blood thinners.

63. Local Bee Pollen Chewables

Train the body to tolerate local allergens with this daily bite.

What It's For:
Bee pollen collected in your area may help your body adapt to the local pollen environment, reducing sensitivity over time.

Ingredients:
- Local, raw bee pollen granules
- Raw honey (optional)
- Mini silicone molds (optional)

Instructions:
1. Press small spoonfuls of bee pollen (and honey, if desired) into molds.
2. Chill until firm. Store in the fridge.

How to Use:

Start with just a few granules per day and gradually increase to ½-1 tsp daily.

Not safe for those with bee or pollen allergies.

64. Chamomile & Rooibos Allergy Tea

A soothing, antihistamine-rich tea for irritated eyes, throat, and skin.

What It's For:
Chamomile is anti-inflammatory and calming, while rooibos is rich in antioxidants and supports respiratory ease.

Ingredients:
- 1 tsp dried chamomile flowers
- 1 tsp rooibos tea
- Optional: pinch of fennel seed or lemon balm

Instructions:
1. Steep herbs in boiling water for 10-15 minutes.
2. Strain and enjoy warm or chilled.

How to Use:

Drink 1-3 cups daily during allergy season.

Avoid chamomile if allergic to ragweed.

65. Nasal Rinse with Goldenseal

Clears nasal passages and reduces inflammation at the source.

What It's For:
A saline rinse flushes out pollen and dust, while goldenseal acts as a natural antimicrobial and inflammation soother.

Ingredients:
- 1 cup sterile or boiled water (cooled)
- ¼ tsp sea salt
- ¼ tsp baking soda
- 10-15 drops goldenseal tincture (optional)
- Neti pot or nasal spray bottle

Instructions:
1. Mix ingredients until fully dissolved.
2. Pour into your neti pot or bottle.

How to Use:

Rinse each nostril 1-2 times daily during allergy flare-ups.

Discard leftovers after 24 hours. Not for use in young children.

66. Lemon-Basil Decongestant Shot

A refreshing, sinus-clearing mini tonic to open the airways.

What It's For:

Basil has anti-inflammatory properties and supports respiratory health, while lemon and apple cider vinegar help clear mucus and balance histamine response.

Ingredients:

- Juice of 1 lemon
- 1 tbsp chopped fresh basil (or 1 tsp dried)
- 1 tbsp apple cider vinegar
- 1 tsp raw honey (optional)
- Small pinch of cayenne (optional)

Instructions:

1. Muddle basil in the lemon juice and vinegar.
2. Strain and add honey and cayenne if using.
3. Shake or stir well.

How to Use:

Take 1 small shot (1-2 oz) once or twice daily during allergy season.

---

67. Elderflower & Peppermint Tea

A cooling, soothing herbal tea for sinus pressure and congestion.

What It's For:

Elderflower acts as a gentle decongestant and anti-inflammatory, while peppermint helps open airways and reduce pressure in the sinuses.

Ingredients:

- 1 tsp dried elderflowers
- 1 tsp dried peppermint
- 1½ cups boiling water

Instructions:

1. Steep herbs for 10-15 minutes.
2. Strain and enjoy warm or cool.

How to Use:

Drink up to 3 cups daily for allergy congestion or pressure relief.

Also helpful during colds with sinus involvement.

68. Natural Antihistamine Salve

A gentle balm to calm itchy skin, hives, or allergy flare-ups.

What It's For:
This topical salve combines soothing, antihistamine-rich herbs like plantain and chamomile to ease irritated, itchy skin from allergies or bug bites.

Ingredients:

- 1 tbsp dried plantain leaf
- 1 tbsp dried chamomile
- ½ cup olive oil
- 1 tbsp beeswax
- Optional: 2 drops lavender essential oil

Instructions:

1. Infuse herbs in oil over low heat for 30 minutes or using the sun infusion method.
2. Strain, then melt beeswax into the oil.
3. Stir in essential oil and pour into tins.

How to Use:

Apply to itchy, inflamed skin as needed. Store in a cool place.

69. Turmeric & Ginger Shot

A powerful anti-inflammatory shot for allergy-related inflammation.

What It's For:
Turmeric and ginger work together to calm systemic inflammation, reduce histamine response, and support immune balance.

Ingredients:

- 1 tbsp fresh grated turmeric (or 1 tsp ground)
- 1 tbsp fresh grated ginger
- Juice of 1 orange or 2 lemons
- Pinch of black pepper (to enhance turmeric absorption)
- 1 tsp raw honey (optional)

Instructions:

1. Blend all ingredients with ½ cup water.
2. Strain and pour into a small jar or shot bottles.

How to Use:

Take 1-2 oz daily as a preventive or as-needed tonic during flare-ups.
Not recommended for those on blood thinners or during pregnancy without guidance.

---

70. Hay Fever Eye Soothing Compress

A cooling herbal compress to relieve itchy, watery, allergy-prone eyes.

What It's For:

Chamomile and calendula calm inflammation and reduce itchiness, while the cold compress helps soothe irritation and puffiness.

Ingredients:

- 1 tsp dried chamomile
- 1 tsp dried calendula
- 1 cup boiling water
- 2 clean cotton pads or soft cloths

Instructions:

1. Steep herbs in water for 10 minutes. Strain well and cool completely.
2. Soak cotton pads in the tea, then place over closed eyes for 10-15 minutes.

How to Use:

Use once or twice daily during allergy flares.
Always strain very well — herbal particles should not enter the eyes.

MANAGING BLOOD SUGAR AND DIABETES

Managing blood sugar isn't just about restriction — it's about *nourishment.* It's about giving the body tools to regulate itself gently and naturally, without spikes and crashes. Herbal remedies can support insulin sensitivity, reduce sugar cravings, and help maintain stable energy throughout the day. This section includes teas, tonics, and foods that work with your body — not against it — and can be layered alongside medical care and healthy habits. While herbs aren't a replacement for professional guidance, they offer meaningful support, especially when used consistently and intentionally.

71. Cinnamon & Gymnema Tea

A warming tea that curbs cravings and supports insulin sensitivity.

What It's For:

Cinnamon helps lower fasting blood sugar, and gymnema is known as the "sugar destroyer" for its ability to block sugar absorption and reduce cravings.

Ingredients:

- 1 cinnamon stick or 1 tsp ground cinnamon
- 1 tsp dried gymnema leaf
- 1½ cups boiling water

Instructions:

1. Simmer cinnamon for 10 minutes, then add gymnema and steep for another 5-10 minutes.
2. Strain and sip warm.

How to Use:

Drink once or twice daily, especially after meals.

Consult your provider before using with insulin or glucose-lowering medications.

72. Bitter Melon Capsules

A concentrated form of a traditional blood sugar-lowering food.

What It's For:

Bitter melon may help reduce blood sugar levels by mimicking insulin. It's traditionally used in Ayurvedic and Chinese medicine for blood sugar support.

Ingredients:

- Dried bitter melon powder
- Empty capsules (size 00)

Instructions:

1. Fill capsules with powdered bitter melon.
2. Store in a sealed glass jar.

How to Use:

Take 1-2 capsules with meals, once or twice daily.

Start slow, as bitter melon is very potent. Not recommended during pregnancy.

73. Mulberry Leaf Infusion

A gentle daily tea to support healthy glucose absorption.

What It's For:

Mulberry leaves help inhibit the absorption of sugars in the gut, supporting more balanced post-meal blood sugar levels.

Ingredients:

- 1 tbsp dried mulberry leaf
- 1½ cups boiling water

Instructions:

1. Steep leaves in boiling water for 10-15 minutes.
2. Strain and enjoy warm or over ice.

How to Use:

Drink 1-2 cups daily, especially before or after carbohydrate-rich meals.

Avoid during pregnancy or when taking insulin without medical supervision.

74. Fenugreek Seed Porridge

A nourishing breakfast that supports digestion and lowers blood sugar spikes.

What It's For:

Fenugreek seeds are high in fiber and compounds that help manage blood glucose and cholesterol. This porridge is especially helpful in the morning when blood sugar tends to rise.

Ingredients:

- 1 tbsp whole fenugreek seeds (soaked overnight)
- ½ cup rolled oats or millet
- 1 cup plant-based milk or water
- Cinnamon and nutmeg to taste

Instructions:

1. Rinse soaked fenugreek and simmer with oats and milk until soft.
2. Add warming spices and sweeten lightly if needed (stevia or monk fruit suggested).

How to Use:

Enjoy as a balanced, blood sugar-friendly breakfast.

75. Berberine-Rich Root Tonic

A powerful herbal tonic for blood sugar, metabolism, and gut health.

What It's For:
Berberine is found in herbs like Oregon grape root, barberry, and goldenseal. It supports healthy blood glucose, insulin response, and even cholesterol balance.

Ingredients:

- 1 tbsp dried Oregon grape root or barberry
- 1 cup vodka or apple cider vinegar
- Glass jar with lid

Instructions:

1. Combine root and liquid in a jar.
2. Steep for 3-4 weeks, shaking every few days.
3. Strain and bottle.

How to Use:

Take ½ to 1 dropperful before meals, 1-2 times daily.

Do not use long-term without supervision. Avoid during pregnancy.

76. Apple Cider Vinegar & Cinnamon Tonic

A simple pre-meal tonic to help lower post-meal glucose spikes.

What It's For:
ACV helps slow the breakdown of starches, while cinnamon improves insulin sensitivity. Together, they make a powerful duo for metabolic health.

Ingredients:

- 1 tbsp raw apple cider vinegar
- ½ tsp ground cinnamon
- 1 cup warm or room temperature water
- Optional: squeeze of lemon or a dash of stevia

Instructions:

1. Mix ingredients in a glass and stir well.
2. Sip slowly 10-15 minutes before meals.

How to Use:

Take 1-2 times daily before main meals.

Rinse mouth after use to protect tooth enamel.

77. Herbal Blood Sugar Chai

A spicy, rich blend of herbs that regulate sugar and warm digestion.

What It's For:

This warming chai features blood sugar-friendly herbs like cinnamon, fenugreek, and ginger — making it both a healing drink and a cozy ritual.

Ingredients:

- 1 tsp cinnamon chips or powder
- ½ tsp fenugreek seeds
- ½ tsp dried ginger
- ¼ tsp cardamom
- 1 cup water + ½ cup milk (dairy or plant-based)

Instructions:

1. Simmer herbs in water for 10-15 minutes.
2. Add milk and gently warm.
3. Strain and sweeten lightly if desired.

How to Use:

Enjoy mid-morning or afternoon as a caffeine-free energy stabilizer.

78. Hibiscus-Cinnamon Cold Brew

A refreshing antioxidant-rich drink that also helps reduce blood pressure and sugar levels.

What It's For:

Hibiscus lowers blood pressure and blood sugar, while cinnamon offers insulin support. This cold brew is tangy, cooling, and ideal for warmer seasons.

Ingredients:

- 1 tbsp dried hibiscus petals
- ½ tsp cinnamon chips or powder
- 2 cups cold water

Instructions:

1. Combine all ingredients in a jar and steep in the fridge for 4-6 hours.
2. Strain and serve over ice.

How to Use:

Drink 1-2 cups per day.

Avoid hibiscus during pregnancy or with very low blood pressure.

79. Coriander-Cardamom Blood Sugar Mix

A warming seed-based blend to support digestion and stable glucose.

What It's For:

Coriander seeds support liver and insulin function, and cardamom soothes digestion while supporting metabolic balance.

Ingredients:

- 1 tsp coriander seeds
- ½ tsp cardamom seeds or powder
- Optional: pinch of fennel or cinnamon

Instructions:

1. Grind seeds into a powder or lightly crush.
2. Mix into warm water, tea, or sprinkle on meals.

How to Use:

Use ½-1 tsp per day. Great in teas, smoothies, or sprinkled on porridge.

Can also be brewed as a simple tea with boiling water.

80. Insulin Plant Green Smoothie

A vibrant, chlorophyll-rich smoothie with blood sugar benefits.

What It's For:

The "insulin plant" (*Costus igneus*) may help lower glucose levels naturally. Blended with greens and fiber, it becomes a refreshing, blood sugar-balancing smoothie.

Ingredients:

- 2-3 fresh insulin plant leaves (or 1 tsp powdered form)
- ½ cup cucumber
- ½ green apple
- 1 handful spinach or kale
- Juice of ½ lemon
- 1 cup water or coconut water

Instructions:

1. Blend all ingredients until smooth.
2. Drink immediately for freshness and potency.

How to Use:

Drink once daily, preferably in the morning or before meals.

Check with your provider before use if you're on diabetes medications.

PAIN RELIEF AND INFLAMMATION REDUCTION

Pain is a message from the body — a signal to slow down, tend inward, and support healing. Whether it's an old injury, achy joints, or inflammation from daily wear and tear, herbal remedies offer meaningful relief without the long list of side effects that often accompany conventional options. This section focuses on time-tested herbs and preparations that ease pain, reduce swelling, and support long-term healing from the inside out. From golden pastes to tinctures and topical salves, these remedies are accessible, effective, and kind to your system.

---

81. Turmeric & Black Pepper Golden Paste

A daily anti-inflammatory blend to ease joint pain and stiffness.

What It's For:

Turmeric is a potent anti-inflammatory herb. Black pepper boosts its absorption, while coconut oil adds fat to further enhance bioavailability.

Ingredients:

- ¼ cup turmeric powder
- ½ tsp ground black pepper
- ½ cup water (plus more as needed)
- 2 tbsp coconut oil

Instructions:

1. In a saucepan, combine turmeric and water.
2. Simmer over low heat for 7-10 minutes, stirring to create a paste.
3. Stir in black pepper and coconut oil. Let cool.
4. Store in a jar in the fridge for up to 2 weeks.

How to Use:

Take ½-1 tsp daily in tea, warm milk, or smoothies.

Not for use during pregnancy or with blood thinners unless supervised.

82. White Willow Bark Tea

Nature's original aspirin—for headaches, cramps, and inflammation.

What It's For:
White willow bark contains salicin, a compound similar to aspirin, making it helpful for pain, fever, or inflammation.

Ingredients:

- 1 tsp dried white willow bark
- 1½ cups water

Instructions:

1. Simmer bark gently in water for 10-15 minutes.
2. Strain and sip warm.

How to Use:

Drink 1-2 cups as needed for pain relief.

Avoid if allergic to aspirin, pregnant, or taking blood thinners.

83. Arnica & Cayenne Salve

A topical remedy for sore muscles, bruises, and deep aches.

What It's For:
Arnica reduces inflammation and bruising, while cayenne boosts circulation and eases nerve pain. A powerful combo for topical relief.

Ingredients:

- ½ cup arnica-infused oil
- ½ tsp cayenne powder
- ¼ cup beeswax
- Optional: 5 drops wintergreen or peppermint essential oil

Instructions:

1. Gently warm infused oil and beeswax until melted.
2. Stir in cayenne and essential oils.
3. Pour into tins and allow to cool.

How to Use:

Rub onto sore areas 2-3 times daily.

Do not apply to broken skin. Wash hands after use.

84. Ginger Compress for Joint Pain

A warming herbal compress to stimulate circulation and relieve stiffness.

What It's For:
Ginger increases blood flow and reduces inflammation, making it ideal for stiff joints, arthritis, and chronic pain.

Ingredients:

- 2 tbsp fresh grated ginger (or 1 tbsp dried)
- 4 cups hot water
- Clean cloth or towel

Instructions:

1. Steep ginger in hot water for 10 minutes.
2. Soak cloth in the infusion, wring out, and apply to affected area.
3. Cover with a dry towel to retain heat.

How to Use:

Apply for 20-30 minutes, once or twice daily.

85. Boswellia Tincture

A powerful internal remedy for inflammation and joint degeneration.

What It's For:
Boswellia (frankincense resin) is traditionally used for arthritis, joint inflammation, and chronic pain. It works by inhibiting inflammatory enzymes in the body.

Ingredients:

- 2 tbsp powdered boswellia resin
- 1 cup high-proof alcohol (vodka or brandy)

Instructions:

1. Combine ingredients in a jar and steep for 4-6 weeks.
2. Shake regularly. Strain and store in a dropper bottle.

How to Use:

Take ½ to 1 dropperful once or twice daily.

Consult your practitioner if pregnant or on medications.

86. Devil's Claw Capsules

An herbal supplement for chronic joint pain and inflammation.

What It's For:
Devil's claw is a traditional remedy from Southern Africa known for reducing pain and stiffness, especially in arthritis and back pain.

Ingredients:
- Dried devil's claw root powder
- Size 00 empty capsules
- Capsule machine (optional)

Instructions:
1. Fill capsules with powdered devil's claw.
2. Store in a labeled jar in a cool, dry place.

How to Use:

Take 1-2 capsules daily with food.

Avoid during pregnancy or with ulcers. Consult a provider for long-term use.

87. Comfrey & Lavender Massage Oil

A nourishing oil to soothe sore muscles, joints, and inflammation.

What It's For:
Comfrey supports tissue repair and joint healing, while lavender calms the nervous system and eases tension.

Ingredients:
- ½ cup comfrey-infused oil
- 10 drops lavender essential oil
- Optional: 1 tbsp arnica-infused oil for added support

Instructions:
1. Combine all oils in a glass bottle.
2. Shake gently to mix.

How to Use:

Massage into sore muscles, joints, or stiff areas 1-2 times daily.

Do not apply comfrey to broken skin or open wounds.

88. Clove Oil Tooth Pain Relief

A potent, fast-acting remedy for toothaches and gum inflammation.

What It's For:
Clove oil contains eugenol, a natural anesthetic and antiseptic. It's ideal for short-term relief of dental pain or sore gums.

Ingredients:

- 2-3 drops clove essential oil
- 1 tsp carrier oil (coconut or olive)
- Cotton swab or small cloth

Instructions:

1. Dilute clove oil with carrier oil.
2. Dip a swab or cloth and apply directly to the painful area.

How to Use:

Use 1-2 times daily as needed.

Do not use undiluted. Not recommended for children under 12.

89. Meadowsweet Anti-Inflammatory Tea

A gentle, aspirin-like tea for chronic pain, headaches, or inflammation.

What It's For:
Meadowsweet contains salicylates, making it helpful for tension headaches, sore muscles, and inflammatory conditions.

Ingredients:

- 1 tsp dried meadowsweet
- 1½ cups hot water
- Optional: lemon balm or chamomile for extra calming effect

Instructions:

1. Steep herbs in hot water for 10-15 minutes.
2. Strain and enjoy warm.

How to Use:

Drink 1-2 cups daily for pain support.

Avoid if allergic to aspirin or during pregnancy.

90. Frankincense & Myrrh Joint Balm

A deeply grounding salve for chronic joint pain and inflammation.

What It's For:

Frankincense and myrrh are traditional resins known for anti-inflammatory, circulatory, and analgesic properties — perfect for arthritis and deep-seated tension.

Ingredients:

- ½ cup olive or jojoba oil
- 1 tbsp frankincense resin
- 1 tbsp myrrh resin
- ¼ cup beeswax
- Optional: 5 drops copaiba or rosemary essential oil

Instructions:

1. Gently infuse resins in oil over low heat for 2-3 hours.
2. Strain, then melt beeswax into the oil.
3. Add essential oils and pour into balm tins.

How to Use:

Massage into joints and sore areas 1-2 times daily.

Store in a cool place. Avoid open wounds or sensitive skin.

Chapter 5

APOTHECARY ON DIFFERENT PARTS OF THE BODY

The body speaks in whispers and signals. A tension in the temples. Dry, irritated skin. An aching back after a long day. These signs aren't just discomforts — they're invitations to connect, care, and nourish from the inside out. In this chapter, we'll explore how to support different parts of the body with intentional, plant-powered remedies that meet us where we are.

Each system of the body — skin, joints, digestion, lungs, reproductive organs — has its own rhythm and needs. And nature offers a rich pharmacy for every one of them. From cooling herbal compresses for tired eyes to salves for cracked heels, from belly-soothing teas to scalp treatments and chest rubs, this chapter is your guide to building a whole-body herbal toolkit.

Instead of thinking of herbalism as one-size-fits-all, we begin to refine. To listen. To say: *my digestion needs warmth*, *my lungs need moisture*, or *my hands need nourishment after a long day in the garden.* It's here that your home apothecary becomes personal — a reflection of your own rhythms, routines, and body wisdom.

We'll organize remedies by body part and body system — so you can easily find what you need, when you need it. You don't need to be an expert to begin. You just need curiosity, a few herbs, and the willingness to care for yourself with intention.

Let's explore how to bring herbal healing to every inch of your being — head to toe, heart to skin, bone to belly.

HERBAL SKINCARE: NATURAL BEAUTY FROM WITHIN

True beauty begins with nourishment — not just of the skin, but of the nervous system, the cells, the senses. Herbal skincare is about more than surface-level results; it's about tuning into what your skin is asking for and offering it real, botanical nourishment. This section is filled with simple, healing recipes to cleanse, restore, and bring out your natural glow — all made with ingredients you can feel good about. Whether you're tending to dryness, dullness, or just craving a moment of self-care, these herbal blends will help you create a skincare ritual that feels grounding, luxurious, and deeply personal.

---

91. Calendula-Rose Face Serum

A gentle, healing oil blend for glowing, balanced skin.

What It's For:
Calendula soothes irritation and supports skin repair, while rose helps hydrate and tone. This serum is especially lovely for dry, sensitive, or mature skin.

Ingredients:

- 2 tbsp calendula-infused oil (like jojoba or sweet almond)
- 1 tbsp rosehip seed oil
- 3 drops rose essential oil (or geranium as a budget-friendly alternative)
- Optional: 1 drop vitamin E oil

Instructions:

1. Combine all ingredients in a small dropper bottle.
2. Shake gently to blend.

How to Use:
Massage 2-3 drops into clean skin at night or under your daily moisturizer.

92. Green Clay Detox Mask

A purifying mask to draw out impurities and rebalance oily or breakout-prone skin.

What It's For:

Green clay is mineral-rich and deeply cleansing. It helps absorb excess oil, clear clogged pores, and leave skin feeling refreshed and toned.

Ingredients:

- 1 tbsp French green clay
- 1 tsp apple cider vinegar or water
- Optional: 1-2 drops tea tree or lavender essential oil

Instructions:

1. Mix clay and liquid to form a paste.
2. Add essential oil if using.

How to Use:

Apply to face, avoiding eyes. Let dry for 5-10 minutes, then rinse with warm water. Use 1-2 times weekly.

93. Turmeric & Honey Brightening Paste

A simple, golden blend for glowing, even-toned skin.

What It's For:

Turmeric reduces redness and supports radiant skin, while honey is naturally antibacterial and deeply hydrating.

Ingredients:

- 1 tsp turmeric powder
- 1 tsp raw honey
- Optional: a few drops milk or yogurt for a creamier texture

Instructions:

1. Mix ingredients into a smooth paste.
2. Apply immediately.

How to Use:

Apply to clean skin and leave on for 10-15 minutes. Rinse thoroughly.

Use caution — turmeric can temporarily stain fair skin or fabrics.

94. Aloe & Lavender Facial Toner

A refreshing, balancing mist to soothe and hydrate throughout the day.

What It's For:

Aloe cools and calms irritated skin, while lavender supports clarity and healing. This toner is gentle enough for daily use on all skin types.

Ingredients:

- ¼ cup aloe vera juice (store-bought or fresh, strained)
- ¼ cup distilled water or rosewater
- 5 drops lavender essential oil
- 1 tsp witch hazel (optional)

Instructions:

1. Combine all ingredients in a small spray bottle.
2. Shake before each use.

How to Use:

Spritz onto clean skin after cleansing or anytime your skin needs a boost.

95. Herbal Facial Steam (Rose, Chamomile, Lavender)

A dreamy, aromatic ritual to open pores and calm the mind.

What It's For:

Facial steaming helps soften skin, release toxins, and open the pores for deeper cleansing. The calming herbs also soothe the senses and reduce inflammation.

Ingredients:

- 1 tbsp dried rose petals
- 1 tbsp dried chamomile
- 1 tbsp dried lavender
- 3-4 cups just-boiled water

Instructions:

1. Place herbs in a heat-safe bowl and pour hot water over them.
2. Lean over the bowl with a towel over your head and breathe deeply for 5-10 minutes.

How to Use:

Follow with a gentle mask or serum. Use weekly or as part of a self-care ritual.

96. Dandelion & Nettle Skin Detox Tea

An internal cleanse to support clear, glowing skin from within.

What It's For:
Both dandelion and nettle support liver detoxification and reduce inflammation, making them powerful allies for acne, dull skin, and hormonal breakouts.

Ingredients:
- 1 tsp dried dandelion leaf or root
- 1 tsp dried nettle leaf
- 2 cups boiling water

Instructions:
1. Steep herbs in boiling water for 15-20 minutes.
2. Strain and enjoy warm or over ice.

How to Use:

Drink 1-2 cups daily for at least two weeks to support clearer skin from within.

97. Sea Buckthorn Glow Balm

A deeply nourishing balm to restore radiance and heal damaged skin.

What It's For:
Sea buckthorn oil is rich in omega fatty acids and antioxidants that support skin regeneration, reduce redness, and promote a healthy glow.

Ingredients:
- 1 tbsp sea buckthorn oil
- 2 tbsp shea butter
- 1 tbsp jojoba oil
- 1 tbsp beeswax

Instructions:
1. Gently melt beeswax and shea butter in a double boiler.
2. Stir in sea buckthorn and jojoba oils.
3. Pour into a small jar and let cool.

How to Use:

Massage a small amount into face or dry patches at night. A little goes a long way!

98. Chamomile-Infused Cleansing Oil

A gentle oil cleanser for sensitive or easily irritated skin.

What It's For:

Chamomile calms inflammation and redness, while oil cleansing helps dissolve makeup, dirt, and excess sebum without stripping the skin.

Ingredients:

- ¼ cup chamomile-infused jojoba or sweet almond oil
- Optional: 2 drops chamomile or lavender essential oil

Instructions:

1. Infuse oil with dried chamomile over low heat or sun-infuse for 1-2 weeks.
2. Strain and store in a glass dropper bottle.

How to Use:

Massage a quarter-sized amount into dry skin. Wipe clean with a warm, damp cloth.

99. Rosemary & Mint Pore-Tightening Mist

A cooling herbal mist to clarify and refresh oily or acne-prone skin.

What It's For:

Rosemary tones the skin and reduces excess oil, while mint cools and refreshes — making this perfect for mid-day spritzes or after workouts.

Ingredients:

- 1 tsp dried rosemary
- 1 tsp dried peppermint
- 1 cup boiling water
- 1 tsp witch hazel (optional)

Instructions:

1. Steep herbs in boiling water for 15 minutes.
2. Strain, cool, and pour into a spray bottle with witch hazel.

How to Use:

Spritz on clean skin, especially in the T-zone, or anytime your skin feels oily or overheated.

100. Plantain & Tea Tree Spot Treatment

A fast-acting herbal remedy for blemishes, bug bites, and small breakouts.

What It's For:

Plantain is anti-inflammatory and draws out impurities, while tea tree oil is antimicrobial and helps dry out blemishes quickly.

Ingredients:

- 1 tbsp plantain-infused oil
- 3-5 drops tea tree essential oil
- Optional: a dab of bentonite clay or aloe gel

Instructions:

1. Mix ingredients and store in a small container.
2. For added power, blend with a pinch of clay or aloe for a creamy texture.

How to Use:

Dab a small amount directly onto blemishes 1-2 times daily.

HAIRCARE SOLUTIONS: NOURISH AND REVITALIZE

Haircare, like skincare, is deeply personal — and the herbs that nourish our roots can often tell a story of tradition, balance, and beauty. Whether you're aiming to stimulate hair growth, soothe an irritated scalp, or bring luster back to tired strands, herbal remedies offer gentle and effective solutions that get to the root of the issue — literally.

This section features time-tested infusions, oils, and rinses that support scalp health, improve hair texture, and strengthen hair from follicle to tip. Free from synthetic chemicals or harsh treatments, these blends let your hair (and you) thrive naturally. With a little intention and consistency, your haircare routine can become a ritual of nourishment and renewal.

101. Rosemary Hair Growth Oil

A stimulating scalp oil to support circulation and follicle health.

What It's For:

Rosemary promotes blood flow to the scalp and may help encourage hair growth and thickness over time.

Ingredients:

- ¼ cup rosemary-infused olive or jojoba oil
- 5 drops rosemary essential oil
- Optional: 3 drops peppermint essential oil (for extra tingle)

Instructions:

1. Blend infused oil with essential oils in a glass bottle.
2. Shake gently to mix.

How to Use:

Massage a few drops into the scalp 2-3 times a week. Leave in for at least 30 minutes or overnight before washing out.

102. Nettle & Horsetail Strengthening Rinse

A mineral-rich herbal rinse to reduce shedding and strengthen hair.

What It's For:

Nettle and horsetail are high in silica and iron, helping to fortify hair strands and reduce breakage.

Ingredients:

- 1 tbsp dried nettle leaf
- 1 tbsp dried horsetail
- 2 cups boiling water

Instructions:

1. Steep herbs in boiling water for 30-45 minutes.
2. Strain and let cool.

How to Use:

After shampooing, pour rinse over hair and massage into scalp. Do not rinse out. Use 1-2 times per week.

103. Aloe & Peppermint Scalp Soother

A cooling gel to calm irritation, itchiness, or scalp inflammation.

What It's For:

Aloe vera hydrates and heals, while peppermint provides cooling relief and stimulates circulation.

Ingredients:

- 2 tbsp fresh or pure aloe vera gel
- 3 drops peppermint essential oil
- Optional: 1 tsp witch hazel (for oily scalps)

Instructions:

1. Mix ingredients in a small bowl or bottle.
2. Store in the fridge for up to 5 days.

How to Use:

Apply directly to scalp after washing or between washes. Massage in and let absorb.

104. Lavender & Argan Deep Conditioner

A luxurious oil blend to hydrate, soften, and protect dry or damaged hair.

What It's For:

Lavender supports scalp balance, and argan oil deeply nourishes dry or frizzy hair while adding shine and softness.

Ingredients:

- 2 tbsp argan oil
- 1 tbsp coconut or avocado oil
- 5 drops lavender essential oil

Instructions:

1. Mix all ingredients in a small jar or bottle.
2. Warm slightly before applying if desired.

How to Use:

Work into hair from mid-length to ends. Wrap in a towel or shower cap and leave on for 30 minutes to overnight. Shampoo thoroughly to rinse.

105. Fermented Rice & Hibiscus Hair Rinse

A traditional strengthening rinse for softness, shine, and smoother strands.

What It's For:

Fermented rice water strengthens hair, reduces breakage, and promotes growth. Hibiscus adds shine and may help with scalp health.

Ingredients:

- ½ cup uncooked rice
- 2 cups water
- 1 tbsp dried hibiscus petals

Instructions:

1. Rinse rice and soak in water for 24-48 hours until lightly fermented.
2. Add hibiscus and steep for 10-15 minutes, then strain.

How to Use:

Pour over hair after washing. Leave on for 5-10 minutes, then rinse with cool water. Use 1-2 times per week.

106. Herbal Dry Shampoo (Sage, Arrowroot, Clay)

A natural powder to refresh roots and absorb excess oil between washes.

What It's For:

Sage helps control oil and supports scalp health, arrowroot absorbs moisture, and clay gently detoxifies. Great for oily or fine hair.

Ingredients:

- 2 tbsp arrowroot powder
- 1 tbsp bentonite or kaolin clay
- 1 tbsp dried sage, finely ground
- Optional: 1 tbsp cocoa powder (for darker hair tones)

Instructions:

1. Mix all ingredients and store in a shaker jar or spice container.
2. Apply with a makeup brush or fingertips to roots.

How to Use:

Dust onto scalp and roots, let sit for a few minutes, then brush through thoroughly.

107. Marshmallow Root Detangling Spray

A slippery, conditioning spray to smooth tangles and hydrate strands.

What It's For:

Marshmallow root is rich in mucilage, creating a natural "slip" that softens and detangles hair without synthetic conditioners.

Ingredients:

- 1 tbsp dried marshmallow root
- 1½ cups hot water
- Optional: 1 tsp aloe vera gel or 2 drops lavender essential oil

Instructions:

1. Steep marshmallow root in hot water for 30-45 minutes.
2. Strain well and mix in optional ingredients. Pour into a spray bottle.

How to Use:

Spritz on damp or dry hair before brushing or styling. Store in fridge for up to one week.

108. Neem & Tea Tree Dandruff Tonic

A powerful herbal remedy to rebalance the scalp and reduce flakes.

What It's For:

Neem is antifungal and supports scalp healing, while tea tree essential oil helps manage dandruff, itchiness, and buildup.

Ingredients:

- 1 tbsp dried neem leaf or 10 drops neem oil
- 1 cup hot water
- 5 drops tea tree essential oil
- Optional: 1 tsp witch hazel

Instructions:

1. Steep neem leaves in hot water for 15-20 minutes.
2. Strain, let cool, and add tea tree oil and witch hazel.
3. Pour into a spray bottle.

How to Use:

Spray directly onto scalp and massage in. Use 2-3 times weekly after shampooing.

109. Rosemary-Vinegar Hair Shine Rinse

A clarifying final rinse that smooths cuticles and boosts shine.

What It's For:

Apple cider vinegar restores pH balance and removes buildup, while rosemary stimulates the scalp and enhances natural luster.

Ingredients:

- 1 tbsp dried rosemary
- 1 cup boiling water
- ¼ cup raw apple cider vinegar

Instructions:

1. Steep rosemary in boiling water for 15 minutes.
2. Strain and mix with vinegar.
3. Pour into a bottle and store in the fridge.

How to Use:

After shampooing, pour rinse over hair. Leave on or rinse lightly with cool water.

110. Coconut-Moringa Scalp Balm

A rich, herbal balm to nourish dry scalps and promote healthy roots.

What It's For:

Coconut oil moisturizes, while moringa is rich in antioxidants and nutrients that support scalp circulation and healing.

Ingredients:

- 2 tbsp coconut oil
- 1 tbsp moringa powder or oil
- Optional: 3 drops peppermint or rosemary essential oil

Instructions:

1. Melt coconut oil gently and stir in moringa.
2. Add essential oils if using. Let cool and solidify in a small jar.

How to Use:

Massage into scalp before washing or leave on overnight as a scalp treatment.

BODYCARE: LUXURIOUS HERBAL TREATMENTS

Herbal bodycare is where healing meets pleasure. These rituals aren't just about moisturized skin or fresh scent — they're about honoring the vessel you move through life in. Whether you're massaging a warming oil into sore muscles, scrubbing away the day's stress, or slipping into a bath infused with plants, these moments offer a return to your body — and to the earth.

This section offers rich, sensory blends made with herbs, oils, and minerals to pamper and restore. Each recipe invites you to slow down, tune in, and care for yourself with intention. Bodycare becomes more than routine — it becomes ritual.

---

111. Whipped Shea Body Butter with Calendula

A deeply moisturizing butter to soothe dry, sensitive, or irritated skin.

What It's For:
Shea butter hydrates and protects, while calendula soothes inflammation and supports skin repair. This blend is rich, healing, and perfect for dry seasons.

Ingredients:

- ½ cup shea butter
- ¼ cup calendula-infused oil (e.g., olive, jojoba)
- 1 tbsp arrowroot powder (optional, reduces greasiness)
- 10 drops lavender or orange essential oil (optional)

Instructions:

1. Melt shea butter and calendula oil together, then chill until firm but not solid.
2. Whip with a hand mixer until fluffy.
3. Stir in arrowroot and essential oils if using. Store in a jar.

How to Use:

Massage into clean skin, especially after bathing.

112. Lavender & Rose Body Oil

A sensual, calming oil for daily self-massage and moisture.

What It's For:
This light, aromatic oil blend softens skin and uplifts the senses. Lavender calms, while rose nourishes both skin and spirit.

Ingredients:

- ¼ cup jojoba or sweet almond oil
- 1 tbsp dried rose petals
- 1 tbsp dried lavender
- Optional: 5 drops rose or lavender essential oil

Instructions:

1. Gently warm oil and herbs in a double boiler or let infuse for 1-2 weeks.
2. Strain and pour into a glass bottle. Add essential oil if desired.

How to Use:

Apply to damp skin after a shower or use as a massage oil.

113. DIY Herbal Deodorant (Tea Tree, Arrowroot, Coconut)

A natural deodorant that's effective, refreshing, and free of toxins.

What It's For:
Coconut oil is antimicrobial, arrowroot helps absorb moisture, and tea tree neutralizes odor-causing bacteria.

Ingredients:

- ¼ cup coconut oil
- ¼ cup arrowroot powder
- 1 tbsp baking soda (reduce for sensitive skin)
- 10 drops tea tree essential oil
- Optional: 5 drops lavender or sage essential oil

Instructions:

1. Mix all ingredients until smooth and creamy.
2. Store in a small jar with a lid.

How to Use:

Apply a pea-sized amount under each arm. Allow to absorb before dressing.

114. Detoxifying Herbal Bath Soak (Epsom, Nettle, Sage)

A mineral-rich soak to release tension, clear toxins, and reset the body.

What It's For:
Epsom salt relaxes muscles and replenishes magnesium. Nettle and sage support detox, circulation, and clarity.

Ingredients:

- 1 cup Epsom salt
- ¼ cup dried nettle
- ¼ cup dried sage
- Optional: 10 drops eucalyptus or rosemary essential oil

Instructions:

1. Blend all ingredients and store in a jar or muslin bag.
2. Add ½-1 cup to a hot bath and soak for 20-30 minutes.

How to Use:

Use weekly for muscle recovery or seasonal detox support.

115. Body Scrub with Coffee, Cinnamon & Clove

A warming, invigorating scrub to exfoliate, boost circulation, and awaken the senses.

What It's For:
Coffee grounds improve skin tone and texture, while cinnamon and clove offer warming, stimulating benefits for tired muscles and dull skin.

Ingredients:

- ½ cup used or fresh coffee grounds
- ¼ cup coconut oil
- 1 tbsp brown sugar
- ½ tsp ground cinnamon
- ¼ tsp ground clove

Instructions:

1. Mix all ingredients into a thick, gritty paste.
2. Store in a jar with a lid (preferably used within 1-2 weeks).

How to Use:

Apply in the shower using circular motions. Rinse thoroughly and follow with body oil or lotion.

116. Herbal Body Wash Base (Castile + Infused Oil)

A gentle, nourishing body wash you can customize with your favorite herbs and essential oils.

What It's For:
Castile soap offers a gentle cleanse, while infused oils bring herbal healing and moisture to your everyday shower ritual.

Ingredients:

- ½ cup unscented liquid Castile soap
- 2 tbsp calendula- or chamomile-infused oil (jojoba, almond, or olive oil)
- 10-15 drops essential oil (lavender, rosemary, or citrus)

Instructions:

1. In a pump bottle, combine all ingredients and shake gently.
2. Store in a cool place; shake before each use.

How to Use:

Use daily as a gentle body cleanser. Safe for most skin types, including sensitive skin.

---

117. Juniper & Ginger Cellulite Massage Blend

A warming, stimulating oil to boost circulation and tone the skin.

What It's For:
Juniper and ginger improve lymphatic flow and circulation, helping to reduce fluid retention and support firmer skin over time.

Ingredients:

- ¼ cup grapeseed or sweet almond oil
- 5 drops juniper berry essential oil
- 5 drops ginger essential oil
- 5 drops grapefruit essential oil (optional)

Instructions:

1. Combine oils in a glass bottle.
2. Shake to blend before each use.

How to Use:

Massage into thighs, hips, or arms in circular, upward motions 1-2 times daily.

118. Minty Cooling Foot Spray

A refreshing spray for tired, hot, or swollen feet—perfect for summer or long days on your feet.

What It's For:
Peppermint cools and invigorates, while witch hazel and aloe soothe and tone.

Ingredients:
- ¼ cup witch hazel
- 2 tbsp aloe vera juice or gel
- 10 drops peppermint essential oil
- Optional: 5 drops tea tree or eucalyptus essential oil

Instructions:
1. Mix ingredients in a small spray bottle.
2. Shake well before each use. Store in the fridge for extra cooling.

How to Use:

Spritz directly onto clean feet and ankles. Use anytime for instant relief.

119. Chamomile & Honey Body Lotion Bar

A soothing, solid moisturizer for sensitive or dry skin.

What It's For:
Chamomile calms inflammation, and honey locks in moisture. This bar melts into the skin with body heat, offering long-lasting hydration.

Ingredients:
- ¼ cup beeswax
- ¼ cup shea or cocoa butter
- ¼ cup chamomile-infused oil
- 1 tsp raw honey (optional)

Instructions:
1. Melt beeswax and butter together, then stir in oil and honey.
2. Pour into silicone molds or small tins. Let cool completely.

How to Use:

Rub directly onto dry skin after bathing. Store in a cool place between uses.

120. Frankincense Body Cream for Dry Skin

A rich, healing cream for deep nourishment and skin renewal.

What It's For:
Frankincense supports skin repair and elasticity, while the creamy base hydrates and protects. Ideal for mature or very dry skin.

Ingredients:
- ¼ cup shea butter
- 2 tbsp avocado or almond oil
- 1 tbsp aloe vera gel
- 10 drops frankincense essential oil

Instructions:
1. Melt shea butter and oil, then allow to cool slightly.
2. Stir in aloe and essential oil.
3. Whip until fluffy and store in a glass jar.

How to Use:
Massage into dry areas daily, especially after bathing.

BRAIN HEALTH: ENHANCING MEMORY AND COGNITIVE FUNCTION

Our brains are constantly processing, solving, remembering, and navigating — often without rest. In today's overstimulated world, it's easy to feel foggy, forgetful, or mentally drained. But nature offers powerful allies to support focus, memory, mental stamina, and long-term cognitive vitality.

This section highlights herbs and fungi traditionally used to support brain health — from quick-acting aromatic blends to deeper tonics that nourish brain function over time. Whether you need to sharpen focus, lift mental fog, or simply feel more alert and grounded, these remedies invite you to care for your mind in a gentle, sustainable way.

121. Ginkgo Biloba Memory Tincture

A traditional remedy to support circulation, memory, and mental clarity.

What It's For:
Ginkgo increases blood flow to the brain and may help improve memory and cognitive performance, especially with consistent use.

Ingredients:
- 2 tbsp dried ginkgo biloba leaf
- 1 cup vodka or brandy (80-100 proof)
- Glass jar with lid

Instructions:
1. Combine ginkgo and alcohol in a jar.
2. Steep for 3-4 weeks, shaking occasionally.
3. Strain and store in a dropper bottle.

How to Use:

Take ½-1 dropperful 1-2 times daily.

Not recommended for those on blood thinners or during pregnancy.

122. Rosemary Essential Oil Roll-On for Focus

An on-the-go aromatherapy blend to uplift the mind and sharpen attention.

What It's For:
Rosemary has been shown to enhance memory and alertness through scent alone. This roll-on is perfect for study, work, or mid-day slumps.

Ingredients:
- 10 ml roller bottle
- 10 drops rosemary essential oil
- 5 drops lemon essential oil
- Carrier oil (like fractionated coconut or jojoba)

Instructions:
1. Add essential oils to the bottle, then fill with carrier oil.
2. Shake gently to combine.

How to Use:

Roll onto temples, wrists, or behind ears before focus-heavy tasks.

123. Brahmi & Gotu Kola Brain Tonic Tea

A deeply nourishing daily tea to support clarity, learning, and calm focus.

What It's For:
Brahmi (Bacopa) and gotu kola are revered Ayurvedic herbs known to support memory, reduce mental fatigue, and enhance cognition over time.

Ingredients:
- 1 tsp dried Brahmi
- 1 tsp dried gotu kola
- Optional: pinch of tulsi or lemon balm
- 2 cups hot water

Instructions:
1. Steep herbs in hot water for 10-15 minutes.
2. Strain and sip slowly.

How to Use:

Drink daily for several weeks for long-term support.

Avoid during pregnancy unless guided.

124. Lion's Mane Mushroom Elixir

A creamy, brain-nourishing drink for neuroprotection and focus.

What It's For:
Lion's mane is a nootropic mushroom shown to support memory, nerve regeneration, and cognitive health — especially useful for brain fog or long-term vitality.

Ingredients:
- 1 tsp lion's mane powder (dual-extract recommended)
- 1 cup warm plant milk (almond, oat, etc.)
- ½ tsp cinnamon
- 1 tsp raw honey or maple syrup

Instructions:
1. Blend all ingredients until smooth and frothy.
2. Warm gently on the stove if desired.

How to Use:

Drink daily or several times per week as a brain-boosting latte.

125. Peppermint & Lemon Brain Fog Inhaler

A quick, refreshing pick-me-up for clarity and mental energy.

What It's For:

Peppermint awakens and stimulates the mind, while lemon uplifts the mood and cuts through sluggishness — perfect for mental fatigue or travel.

Ingredients:

- 5 drops peppermint essential oil
- 5 drops lemon essential oil
- 1 blank aromatherapy inhaler (with cotton wick)

Instructions:

1. Drop oils onto the wick and seal in the inhaler.
2. Store in a cool, dry place.

How to Use:

Inhale deeply through the nose during moments of mental fog, tiredness, or low focus.

---

126. Rhodiola Memory Support Capsules

A convenient adaptogenic supplement for focus and mental stamina.

What It's For:

Rhodiola is an adaptogen that enhances memory, mental clarity, and endurance under stress — especially helpful for students or professionals.

Ingredients:

- Rhodiola rosea root powder (standardized or wildcrafted)
- Empty capsules (size 00)
- Capsule machine (optional)

Instructions:

1. Fill capsules with rhodiola powder.
2. Store in a labeled glass jar away from heat and light.

How to Use:

Take 1-2 capsules (about 400-600 mg) in the morning.

Best used in cycles: 3-4 weeks on, 1 week off. Not for use late in the day.

127. Sage Tea for Mental Clarity

A simple, traditional remedy to sharpen the mind and memory.

What It's For:

Sage has long been associated with wisdom — both spiritually and physiologically. It helps improve memory, reduce brain fog, and enhance clarity.

Ingredients:

- 1 tsp dried sage leaves
- 1½ cups boiling water
- Optional: lemon slice or honey

Instructions:

1. Steep sage in hot water for 10 minutes.
2. Strain and sip warm.

How to Use:

Drink 1-2 cups daily for clarity and cognitive support.
Avoid high doses during pregnancy.

---

128. Nootropic Herbal Smoothie Booster (Maca, Ginseng, Cacao)

A potent powder blend to support memory, mood, and energy.

What It's For:

Maca enhances stamina and hormone balance, ginseng supports alertness and stress resilience, and cacao boosts mood and blood flow to the brain.

Ingredients:

- 1 tbsp maca powder
- 1 tsp ginseng powder
- 1 tbsp raw cacao powder
- Optional: 1 tsp lion's mane or ashwagandha powder

Instructions:

1. Blend with your favorite smoothie base: banana, berries, greens, and plant milk.
2. Sweeten to taste and blend until smooth.

How to Use:

Use 1-2 tablespoons per smoothie. Great for mornings or pre-work sessions.

129. Walnut-Rosemary Infused Oil

A culinary and topical oil blend to nourish brain health and circulation.

What It's For:
Walnuts are rich in brain-loving omega-3s, and rosemary improves circulation and alertness. This oil can be used in cooking or gentle scalp massage.

Ingredients:
- ½ cup walnut oil (cold-pressed)
- 2 tbsp dried rosemary
- Optional: 1 garlic clove or pinch of sea salt

Instructions:
1. Gently warm rosemary in walnut oil for 15-20 minutes (do not overheat).
2. Cool, strain, and bottle.

How to Use:

Use in salad dressings, drizzled on veggies, or massage into scalp for circulation.

130. Turmeric-Ginger Brain Support Latte

A warming, anti-inflammatory drink to support cognition and focus.

What It's For:

Turmeric and ginger reduce inflammation that may contribute to brain fog and sluggish thinking, while warming spices stimulate circulation and mental energy.

Ingredients:
- 1 tsp turmeric powder
- ½ tsp fresh or powdered ginger
- ½ tsp cinnamon
- 1 cup plant milk
- 1 tsp honey or maple syrup
- Pinch of black pepper (enhances turmeric absorption)

Instructions:
1. Warm milk and whisk in all ingredients until smooth and frothy.
2. Pour into a mug and sip slowly.

How to Use:

Enjoy daily as a brain-boosting morning or mid-afternoon ritual.

HERBAL REMEDIES FOR HEADACHES AND MIGRAINES

Headaches speak in pulses, aches, and fog — gentle nudges or full-body alarms that something is out of balance. Whether triggered by stress, hormones, inflammation, or tension, headaches and migraines can interrupt your day and steal your clarity. But with the help of herbs, you can build a toolkit of gentle yet effective remedies to relieve pain, calm the nervous system, and reduce frequency over time.

This section offers both fast-acting relief and long-term support — from aromatic roll-ons and compresses to herbal teas and tinctures. These remedies honor the body's signals without harsh interventions and help you reclaim calm, clarity, and peace.

---

131. Chamomile-Lemon Balm Headache Soak

A soothing herbal bath for full-body tension release and head pain relief.

What It's For:
Chamomile calms the body and nervous system, while lemon balm eases stress and uplifts the mood — perfect for tension-related or hormonal headaches.

Ingredients:
- 1 tbsp dried chamomile
- 1 tbsp dried lemon balm
- 1 cup Epsom salts
- Optional: 5 drops lavender essential oil

Instructions:
1. Combine herbs in a muslin bag or steep in boiling water for 15 minutes.
2. Pour infusion and Epsom salts into bathwater.
3. Add essential oil if using.

How to Use:
Soak for 20-30 minutes in a quiet, low-light space. Breathe deeply and rest afterward.

132. Feverfew Migraine Tea

A gentle, preventive tea for those prone to hormonal or vascular migraines.

What It's For:
Feverfew is a well-known herb used to prevent the frequency and intensity of migraines over time — especially effective when taken daily.

Ingredients:

- 1 tsp dried feverfew
- 1 tsp lemon balm or chamomile (optional)
- 1½ cups boiling water

Instructions:

1. Steep herbs in hot water for 10-15 minutes.
2. Strain and sip warm or cool.

How to Use:

Drink once daily for prevention, or at the onset of a migraine.

Not recommended during pregnancy.

---

133. Peppermint Essential Oil Roll-On

A fast, cooling application for tension headaches or sinus pressure.

What It's For:
Peppermint cools and calms tight muscles, eases pressure, and enhances blood flow to the forehead and temples.

Ingredients:

- 10 ml roller bottle
- 8-10 drops peppermint essential oil
- Optional: 2-3 drops eucalyptus or lavender essential oil
- Carrier oil (fractionated coconut, jojoba, or almond)

Instructions:

1. Add essential oils to bottle and fill with carrier oil.
2. Shake gently to blend.

How to Use:

Roll onto temples, back of neck, and behind ears at first sign of headache.

Avoid contact with eyes.

134. Lavender Cold Compress Infusion

A calming compress to ease tension and support nervous system relaxation.

What It's For:
Lavender helps soothe stress-related or hormonal headaches and brings a sense of calm to body and mind.

Ingredients:

- 1 tbsp dried lavender flowers
- 1 cup hot water
- Clean cloth or muslin

Instructions:

1. Steep lavender in hot water for 10 minutes.
2. Strain and cool the infusion.
3. Soak cloth, wring out, and apply to forehead or back of neck.

How to Use:

Apply for 15-20 minutes in a dark, quiet space. Breathe deeply.

135. Skullcap & Passionflower Relaxation Tincture

A calming nervine formula to ease tension headaches and prevent stress-induced migraines.

What It's For:
Skullcap and passionflower help relax the nervous system, ease muscle tension, and support gentle, sustained calm.

Ingredients:

- 1 tbsp dried skullcap
- 1 tbsp dried passionflower
- 1 cup vodka or brandy (80-100 proof)
- Glass jar with lid

Instructions:

1. Combine herbs and alcohol in a jar and seal.
2. Steep for 3-4 weeks, shaking every few days.
3. Strain and store in a dropper bottle.

How to Use:

Take ½-1 dropperful at the onset of tension or before bed.

Not recommended for use during pregnancy.

136. White Willow Bark Tincture

A herbal alternative to aspirin for reducing pain and inflammation.

What It's For:
White willow bark contains salicin, a natural pain-relieving compound. Ideal for tension or inflammatory headaches.

Ingredients:
- 2 tbsp dried white willow bark
- 1 cup vodka or brandy (80-100 proof)
- Glass jar with lid

Instructions:
1. Steep willow bark in alcohol for 3-4 weeks, shaking occasionally.
2. Strain and store in a dropper bottle.

How to Use:
Take ½-1 dropperful at the onset of headache.

Avoid if allergic to aspirin or using blood thinners.

137. Magnesium Balm with Lavender

A topical balm to relieve muscle tension, neck tightness, and promote restful sleep.

What It's For:
Magnesium supports muscle relaxation and reduces nerve-related tension. Lavender calms both the mind and the body.

Ingredients:
- ½ cup magnesium oil (or magnesium chloride flakes + water)
- ¼ cup coconut oil or shea butter
- 10 drops lavender essential oil

Instructions:
1. Gently melt coconut oil if solid, then whisk in magnesium oil.
2. Stir in lavender and store in a jar.

How to Use:
Massage into neck, shoulders, and temples before bed or at headache onset.

138. Basil & Peppermint Tea for Tension

A refreshing tea to ease tension headaches and promote circulation.

What It's For:

Basil and peppermint both support headache relief by reducing inflammation, encouraging blood flow, and relaxing the body.

Ingredients:

- 1 tsp dried basil
- 1 tsp dried peppermint
- 1½ cups hot water

Instructions:

1. Steep herbs in hot water for 10-12 minutes.
2. Strain and enjoy warm.

How to Use:

Drink at the onset of tension or sip throughout the day to prevent stress-related headaches.

139. Migrastick Roller with Eucalyptus & Lavender

A portable, quick-acting blend to relieve pressure and cool the forehead.

What It's For:

This blend provides instant relief through cooling, circulation-boosting, and calming essential oils. Ideal for migraines, sinus pressure, or tension headaches.

Ingredients:

- 5 drops eucalyptus essential oil
- 5 drops lavender essential oil
- Optional: 2 drops peppermint
- Carrier oil (like fractionated coconut)
- 10 ml roller bottle

Instructions:

1. Add essential oils to roller bottle, fill with carrier oil.
2. Shake gently before each use.

How to Use:

Roll onto temples, base of neck, and across forehead. Use as needed for relief.

140. Ginger-Turmeric Headache Shot

A potent, anti-inflammatory blend to reduce pain and digestive-related headaches.

What It's For:

Ginger and turmeric help reduce inflammation, ease nausea, and relieve tension — especially when headaches stem from digestion or stress.

Ingredients:

- 1 tbsp fresh grated ginger
- 1 tsp turmeric powder or 1-inch fresh turmeric
- Juice of 1 lemon
- Pinch of black pepper
- 1 tsp raw honey
- ½ cup water

Instructions:

1. Blend or whisk ingredients until smooth.
2. Strain if desired. Drink immediately.

How to Use:

Take at first sign of headache, or use preventatively during high-stress periods.

GUT HEALTH AND DIGESTION SUPPORT

The gut is more than just a digestive organ — it's a foundation for energy, mood, immunity, and overall balance. When digestion is off, everything else can feel off too. Fortunately, herbs offer a wide range of support, from calming inflammation and easing bloating to stimulating bile flow and strengthening the gut lining.

This section brings together herbal teas, tonics, and soothing drinks that gently support your body's natural digestive rhythms. Whether you're experiencing sluggish digestion, acid discomfort, or simply want to care for your microbiome with intention, these remedies help restore harmony from the inside out — one sip, one herb at a time.

141. Fennel & Peppermint Digestive Tea

A carminative blend to ease bloating, gas, and post-meal heaviness.

What It's For:

Fennel relaxes intestinal muscles and reduces cramping, while peppermint soothes inflammation and helps move digestion along.

Ingredients:

- 1 tsp crushed fennel seeds
- 1 tsp dried peppermint
- 1½ cups boiling water

Instructions:

1. Steep herbs in boiling water for 10-15 minutes.
2. Strain and enjoy warm after meals.

How to Use:

Drink 1-2 cups daily or after heavy meals.

Avoid peppermint during severe reflux.

142. Ginger Bitters Digestive Tonic

A zesty, activating blend to jumpstart sluggish digestion.

What It's For:

Bitter herbs like ginger and orange peel stimulate digestive secretions and improve bile flow, helping with bloating, appetite loss, and slow digestion.

Ingredients:

- 1 tbsp dried ginger root
- 1 tbsp dried orange peel
- 1 tsp dandelion root
- 1 cup vodka or apple cider vinegar

Instructions:

1. Combine herbs and liquid in a glass jar.
2. Steep for 2-4 weeks, shaking occasionally.
3. Strain and store in a dropper bottle.

How to Use:

Take ½-1 dropperful 15-30 minutes before meals.

143. Lemon Balm Carminative Elixir

A sweet, aromatic blend to ease gas, tension, and digestive discomfort.

What It's For:
Lemon balm calms the nerves and gut, while carminative herbs like fennel and ginger relieve bloating and cramping.

Ingredients:

- 2 tbsp dried lemon balm
- 1 tbsp fennel seed
- 1 tbsp dried ginger
- 1 cup brandy or vodka
- 2-4 tbsp raw honey (to taste)

Instructions:

1. Combine herbs and alcohol in a jar.
2. Steep for 3-4 weeks, shaking occasionally.
3. Strain, then stir in honey to create a sweet elixir.

How to Use:

Take ½-1 tsp after meals for digestive ease and gentle relaxation.
Avoid large doses during early pregnancy.

---

144. Dandelion & Chicory Liver-Gut Support

A gently bitter, coffee-like brew to support detox and digestion together.

What It's For:
Dandelion and chicory both stimulate bile flow, support liver function, and help break down fats and proteins more effectively.

Ingredients:

- 1 tsp roasted dandelion root
- 1 tsp roasted chicory root
- 2 cups water

Instructions:

1. Simmer roots in water for 15-20 minutes.
2. Strain and enjoy warm — plain or with milk and honey.

How to Use:

Drink before meals or in the morning as a digestive wake-up.

145. Aloe Vera Digestive Smoothie

A hydrating blend to soothe inflammation and support regularity.

What It's For:
Aloe vera cools and calms the gut, supports elimination, and may ease occasional constipation or irritation.

Ingredients:
- ¼ cup fresh aloe vera gel (inner fillet only)
- ½ banana
- ½ cup cucumber
- 1 cup coconut water or plain water
- Optional: mint or ginger for flavor

Instructions:
1. Blend all ingredients until smooth.
2. Drink immediately for best benefits.

How to Use:

Enjoy 2-3 times per week or during digestive flare-ups.
Always use food-grade, properly prepared aloe (inner gel only, not latex).

146. Apple Cider Vinegar Herbal Tummy Tonic

A simple, pre-meal tonic to activate digestion and reduce bloating.

What It's For:
Apple cider vinegar stimulates digestive enzymes and bile flow, while herbs like mint and chamomile reduce discomfort and soothe the gut.

Ingredients:
- ¼ cup raw apple cider vinegar
- 1 tbsp dried mint
- 1 tbsp dried chamomile
- Optional: 1 tsp raw honey

Instructions:
1. Steep herbs in vinegar for 1-2 weeks, shaking daily.
2. Strain and store in a glass bottle.

How to Use:

Take 1 tsp in water 10-15 minutes before meals.

147. Licorice Root & Marshmallow Tea

A demulcent, gut-coating tea for acid reflux, ulcers, or sensitive digestion.

What It's For:

Licorice and marshmallow are both soothing to inflamed or irritated tissues. Together, they create a deeply healing tea for leaky gut, GERD, and discomfort.

Ingredients:

- 1 tsp dried licorice root
- 1 tsp dried marshmallow root
- 2 cups cool water

Instructions:

1. Place herbs in water and allow to steep (cold infusion) for 4-6 hours or overnight.
2. Strain and gently warm if desired.

How to Use:

Drink ½ cup before meals or at symptom onset.

Use deglycyrrhizinated licorice (DGL) or avoid long-term use with high blood pressure.

148. Slippery Elm Mucilage Drink

A soothing, protective remedy for acid reflux, ulcers, and inflamed gut lining.

What It's For:

Slippery elm is rich in mucilage that coats and protects the digestive tract, easing discomfort from heartburn, leaky gut, or IBS.

Ingredients:

- 1 tsp slippery elm powder
- 1 cup warm water or almond milk
- Optional: dash of cinnamon or honey

Instructions:

1. Whisk powder into warm (not hot) liquid until smooth.
2. Let sit 5-10 minutes to thicken slightly.

How to Use:

Drink slowly once or twice daily on an empty stomach.

Take separately from medications or supplements (it can affect absorption).

149. Gut-Healing Bone Broth with Herbs

A mineral-rich, collagen-packed broth to restore the gut lining and reduce inflammation.

What It's For:

Bone broth contains gelatin, amino acids, and minerals to nourish the gut, while herbs like thyme, bay, and rosemary offer antimicrobial and anti-inflammatory support.

Ingredients:

- 2-3 lbs bones (chicken, beef, or fish)
- 10 cups water
- 2 tbsp apple cider vinegar
- 1 tsp each dried thyme, rosemary, bay leaf
- Optional: garlic, onion, ginger

Instructions:

1. Simmer all ingredients on low for 12-24 hours.
2. Strain and store in jars or freeze.

How to Use:

Sip 1-2 cups daily, especially on an empty stomach or during gut healing protocols.

150. Triphala Blend for Digestive Regularity

A traditional Ayurvedic formula for gentle cleansing and long-term gut balance.

What It's For:

Triphala combines three fruits (amla, haritaki, bibhitaki) to support elimination, improve absorption, and balance the digestive fire without harsh laxatives.

Ingredients:

- ½ tsp triphala powder
- ½ cup warm water

Instructions:

1. Stir powder into water and let sit 5 minutes.
2. Stir again and drink before bed.

How to Use:

Take nightly for regularity and long-term digestive tone.

May take 1-2 weeks of consistent use for best results.

EYE HEALTH AND VISION SUPPORT

Our eyes work hard — filtering light, reading screens, navigating the world from morning to night. Over time, they become fatigued, strained, or dry, and vision can gradually shift. Herbal remedies can offer both soothing relief and deeper nourishment for eye health, thanks to antioxidants, cooling compresses, and herbal infusions that support circulation, reduce inflammation, and protect delicate eye tissues.

This section brings together time-honored formulas and simple, natural solutions to help keep your vision sharp and your eyes comfortable. Whether you're soothing tired eyes, looking to protect vision as you age, or supporting your system from within, these remedies remind us to slow down and see the world — and ourselves — with clarity and care.

---

151. Eyebright Eye Wash

A classic herbal rinse for itchy, irritated, or allergy-prone eyes.

What It's For:
Eyebright (Euphrasia) is a traditional herb for relieving redness, inflammation, and irritation in the eyes — especially helpful during allergy season or screen strain.

Ingredients:

- 1 tsp dried eyebright
- 1 cup distilled or boiled (cooled) water
- Optional: pinch of sea salt for saline effect

Instructions:

1. Steep eyebright in hot water for 10-15 minutes.
2. Strain *very* well using cheesecloth or a fine filter.
3. Let cool completely.

How to Use:

Use in a sterile eye cup or apply gently with cotton pads. Discard after 24 hours.

152. Carrot & Turmeric Vision Juice

A bright, nutrient-rich juice to support eye health from within.

What It's For:
Carrots provide beta-carotene (vitamin A), while turmeric offers anti-inflammatory protection. Lemon and apple add antioxidants and flavor.

Ingredients:

- 2 large carrots
- 1 green apple
- ½ tsp fresh or powdered turmeric
- Juice of ½ lemon
- Pinch of black pepper (for turmeric absorption)

Instructions:

1. Juice or blend all ingredients with a little water.
2. Strain (if desired) and serve immediately.

How to Use:

Drink several times per week for long-term support of eye and skin health.

153. Chamomile Tea Eye Compress

A cooling, calming compress for tired, puffy, or irritated eyes.

What It's For:
Chamomile reduces swelling, soothes irritation, and calms redness — perfect after a long day of screen time or allergies.

Ingredients:

- 1 tsp dried chamomile flowers
- 1 cup hot water
- 2 clean cotton pads

Instructions:

1. Steep chamomile for 10 minutes, then let the tea cool.
2. Soak cotton pads in the cooled tea and place over closed eyes.

How to Use:

Rest with compresses for 10-15 minutes. Repeat as needed.

Always use well-strained tea to avoid particles in eyes.

154. Calendula & Rosehip Eye Serum

A delicate, antioxidant-rich oil to soothe dryness and reduce fine lines.

What It's For:
Calendula softens and calms the skin, while rosehip oil nourishes with vitamins A and C — perfect for nighttime eye care and reducing puffiness.

Ingredients:

- 1 tbsp calendula-infused oil (like jojoba)
- 1 tbsp rosehip seed oil
- 2 drops vitamin E oil (optional)
- 2 drops lavender or chamomile essential oil (optional)

Instructions:

1. Combine all ingredients in a small dropper or roller bottle.
2. Shake gently to mix.

How to Use:

Apply a tiny drop around the orbital bone at night, tapping gently with fingertips. Avoid direct contact with eyes.

---

155. Bilberry Antioxidant Tea

A vision-boosting tea rich in plant compounds that protect and strengthen the eyes.

What It's For:
Bilberries are loaded with anthocyanins, which help improve night vision, strengthen capillaries in the eyes, and support long-term retinal health.

Ingredients:

- 1 tsp dried bilberries or bilberry leaf
- 1 tsp dried hibiscus (optional, for added antioxidants)
- 1½ cups hot water

Instructions:

1. Steep herbs in hot water for 10-15 minutes.
2. Strain and enjoy warm.

How to Use:

Drink 1-2 cups daily for ongoing vision support.

156. Goji Berry Herbal Snack Mix

A sweet-savory trail mix rich in antioxidants, carotenoids, and eye-loving nutrients.

What It's For:
Goji berries are a traditional Chinese herb known for supporting eyesight and longevity. Paired with seeds and herbs, this mix provides a daily dose of eye-nourishing compounds.

Ingredients:
- ½ cup dried goji berries
- ¼ cup pumpkin seeds
- ¼ cup sunflower seeds
- 1 tbsp dried bilberries or blueberries
- 1 tsp dried rosemary or thyme (optional, for savory depth)

Instructions:
1. Combine all ingredients and store in an airtight jar.
2. Mix can be customized with nuts, coconut, or cacao nibs if desired.

How to Use:

Snack by the handful for vision support on the go.

157. Eyebright-Green Tea Rinse

A cooling herbal blend to refresh tired eyes and reduce puffiness.

What It's For:
Eyebright reduces inflammation and green tea provides antioxidants and mild astringent action — great for puffy eyes and redness.

Ingredients:
- 1 tsp dried eyebright
- 1 green tea bag or 1 tsp loose green tea
- 1 cup boiled water

Instructions:
1. Steep both herbs together for 10 minutes.
2. Strain *very well* through cheesecloth. Cool completely.

How to Use:

Use with a compress or sterile eye cup. Keep chilled and use within 24 hours. Avoid direct contact with open or infected eyes.

158. Herbal Omega Oil (Flax, Sea Buckthorn, Borage)

A homemade blend to nourish the eyes, skin, and brain with essential fatty acids.

What It's For:
Omega-rich oils like flax, borage, and sea buckthorn help lubricate the eyes, reduce dryness, and support cellular repair.

Ingredients:
- 2 tbsp cold-pressed flaxseed oil
- 1 tbsp borage seed oil
- 1 tbsp sea buckthorn oil (or rosehip oil)
- Optional: a few drops lemon essential oil for flavor (internal-use safe)

Instructions:
1. Mix oils in a dark glass bottle and refrigerate.
2. Shake gently before each use.

How to Use:

Take 1 tsp daily with meals or add to smoothies/salads.

Use within 4-6 weeks. Store cold and avoid heating.

---

159. Blueberry-Lavender Antioxidant Smoothie

A calming, vision-nourishing blend to protect the eyes from oxidative stress.

What It's For:
Blueberries and lavender offer antioxidants and anti-inflammatory benefits, helping to protect the eyes from light damage and aging.

Ingredients:
- ½ cup frozen blueberries
- 1 banana
- ½ tsp dried lavender flowers (or 1 drop food-grade lavender oil)
- 1 tbsp flax or chia seeds
- 1 cup plant milk

Instructions:
1. Blend all ingredients until smooth and creamy.
2. Serve immediately.

How to Use:

Enjoy 2-3 times per week to support long-term vision health and nervous system calm.

160. Vitamin A Herbal Gummy Bites

A fun, food-based way to deliver carotenoids and herbal eye support — kid- and adult-friendly!

What It's For:

Carrots and mango provide vitamin A precursors, while herbs like goji and calendula add antioxidants that nourish and protect the eyes.

Ingredients:

- ½ cup carrot juice or mango puree
- 2 tbsp strong calendula-goji tea
- 2 tbsp grass-fed gelatin (or agar powder for vegan option)
- 1-2 tbsp honey or maple syrup
- Silicone gummy molds

Instructions:

1. Warm juice and tea gently. Whisk in gelatin until dissolved.
2. Add sweetener and pour into molds.
3. Chill until set (1-2 hours). Store in fridge.

How to Use:

Enjoy 2-3 gummies per day as a delicious vision-boosting supplement.

SUPPORTING LIVER AND KIDNEY HEALTH NATURALLY

Your liver and kidneys work tirelessly — filtering toxins, balancing fluids, processing hormones, and supporting overall vitality. In today's modern world, they face an increasing load from environmental toxins, medications, processed foods, and stress. The good news? Herbs have been used for centuries to help support these vital organs — not through harsh "cleanses," but through gentle, daily nourishment and restoration.

This section offers teas, broths, tonics, and elixirs that naturally stimulate detox pathways, reduce inflammation, and encourage balance. Whether you're coming off a season of stress, supporting hormonal health, or simply wanting to feel lighter and more energized, these herbal allies can help your liver and kidneys do what they do best — heal, clean, and restore from the inside out.

161. Dandelion & Burdock Detox Tea

A classic herbal duo to support liver cleansing, digestion, and skin health.

What It's For:

Dandelion promotes bile flow and detoxification, while burdock helps purify the blood and gently stimulate the kidneys.

Ingredients:

- 1 tsp dried dandelion root
- 1 tsp dried burdock root
- 2 cups water

Instructions:

1. Simmer herbs in water for 15-20 minutes.
2. Strain and sip warm or cool.

How to Use:

Drink 1 cup daily for 1-2 weeks as part of a seasonal reset.

---

162. Milk Thistle Liver Elixir

A sweet, supportive tonic to regenerate and protect liver cells.

What It's For:

Milk thistle contains silymarin, a compound shown to support liver repair and protect against damage from toxins, alcohol, or medication overload.

Ingredients:

- 2 tbsp crushed milk thistle seeds
- 1 cup brandy or vodka
- 2 tbsp raw honey (or to taste)

Instructions:

1. Soak seeds in alcohol for 4-6 weeks, shaking occasionally.
2. Strain and stir in honey. Bottle and label.

How to Use:

Take ½-1 tsp daily before meals or in tea for long-term liver support.

163. Parsley & Lemon Kidney Flush Tonic

A refreshing tonic to encourage hydration, urinary flow, and kidney cleansing.

What It's For:

Parsley is a gentle diuretic and kidney tonic, while lemon supports alkalinity and hydration — perfect for a light daily detox.

Ingredients:

- 1 handful fresh parsley (or 1 tsp dried)
- Juice of ½ lemon
- 1 cup water

Instructions:

1. Blend parsley and lemon juice with water.
2. Strain or drink as-is.

How to Use:

Drink first thing in the morning for 3-5 days for a gentle flush.

Not recommended in large amounts for those with kidney issues without supervision.

164. Nettle Leaf Cleansing Broth

A mineral-rich, gently detoxifying herbal broth for daily nourishment.

What It's For:

Nettle supports kidney function, reduces inflammation, and replenishes depleted minerals — ideal for post-illness, seasonal shifts, or gentle cleansing.

Ingredients:

- 1 tbsp dried nettle leaf
- 1 tbsp dried parsley or dandelion leaf
- 4 cups vegetable or bone broth
- Optional: garlic, celery, ginger

Instructions:

1. Simmer herbs in broth for 20 minutes.
2. Strain or serve with herbs left in for extra nutrients.

How to Use:

Sip 1-2 cups per day for deep nourishment and gentle detox.

165. Turmeric-Ginger Kidney Support Latte

A warming, anti-inflammatory drink that supports kidney circulation and reduces oxidative stress.

What It's For:

Turmeric and ginger reduce inflammation and protect tissues, while black pepper enhances absorption — perfect for long-term kidney resilience.

Ingredients:

- 1 tsp turmeric powder
- ½ tsp grated fresh ginger (or powder)
- 1 cup coconut or almond milk
- Pinch of black pepper
- 1 tsp raw honey (optional)

Instructions:

1. Warm all ingredients in a saucepan over low heat, whisking until smooth.
2. Pour into a mug and enjoy.

How to Use:

Drink 2-3 times per week to reduce inflammation and gently support detox pathways.

166. Juniper Berry Urinary Cleanser

A powerful antimicrobial and diuretic blend for urinary tract health.

What It's For:

Juniper berries help disinfect the urinary tract and stimulate kidney function. Best for short-term use during mild UTI symptoms or water retention.

Ingredients:

- ½ tsp crushed juniper berries
- 1 cup hot water

Instructions:

1. Steep berries for 15 minutes.
2. Strain and sip warm.

How to Use:

Drink once daily for up to 5 days as needed.

Not for use during pregnancy or kidney conditions. Avoid long-term use.

167. Celery Seed & Cornsilk Tea

A gentle urinary tract soother and diuretic for fluid balance and kidney support.

What It's For:

Celery seed supports uric acid elimination and circulation, while cornsilk soothes irritated urinary tissues — ideal for mild retention, puffiness, or UTI prevention.

Ingredients:

- 1 tsp celery seed
- 1 tsp dried cornsilk
- 2 cups boiling water

Instructions:

1. Steep herbs in boiling water for 15-20 minutes.
2. Strain and sip warm or chilled.

How to Use:

Drink up to 2 cups daily for 3-5 days during mild kidney or bladder discomfort.

Avoid during pregnancy or with low blood pressure.

---

168. Schisandra Berry Detox Drops

An adaptogenic tincture to protect the liver and promote whole-body detoxification.

What It's For:

Schisandra is a five-flavor berry used in Traditional Chinese Medicine to support liver health, detox pathways, hormonal balance, and stress resilience.

Ingredients:

- 2 tbsp dried schisandra berries
- 1 cup vodka or brandy
- Optional: 1 tbsp goji berries or orange peel

Instructions:

1. Combine herbs and alcohol in a jar.
2. Steep for 3-4 weeks, shaking regularly.
3. Strain and store in a dropper bottle.

How to Use:

Take ½ dropperful 1-2 times daily for 2-4 weeks during detox seasons.

169. Lemon Balm & Mint Liver Cleanse

A refreshing herbal tea to support gentle liver detox and nervous system calm.

What It's For:
Lemon balm soothes stress and supports the liver energetically, while mint aids digestion and detoxification. This is a gentle reset for body *and* mood.

Ingredients:
- 1 tsp dried lemon balm
- 1 tsp dried peppermint or spearmint
- 1½ cups boiling water

Instructions:
1. Steep herbs for 10-12 minutes.
2. Strain and enjoy hot or over ice.

How to Use:

Drink daily in spring or after periods of heavy eating, stress, or low energy.

170. Goldenrod Diuretic Tea

A gentle, bright yellow herb to reduce water retention and support urinary tract tone.

What It's For:
Goldenrod is known for reducing excess fluid and supporting the kidneys, especially helpful in seasonal allergies, puffiness, or sluggish lymph flow.

Ingredients:
- 1 tsp dried goldenrod aerial parts
- 1½ cups boiling water

Instructions:
1. Steep for 10-15 minutes.
2. Strain and sip warm.

How to Use:

Drink 1 cup daily for up to 7 days during a mild cleanse or lymphatic support routine.

Avoid during pregnancy or with known Asteraceae allergies.

HERBAL APPROACHES TO CARDIOVASCULAR WELLNESS

The heart is more than a muscle — it's the rhythmic center of your entire body. It carries blood, oxygen, and nutrients to every cell, while responding constantly to stress, movement, emotions, and lifestyle. Herbal cardiovascular care is about supporting this vital system with grace — improving circulation, balancing blood pressure, easing inflammation, and promoting long-term heart health.

This section includes herbs and foods known to tone the heart, lower cholesterol, protect blood vessels, and improve overall resilience. Whether you're proactively supporting your heart or navigating an existing concern, these natural allies work best over time — restoring balance gently and sustainably.

---

171. Hawthorn Heart Tonic

A deeply nourishing herbal extract to strengthen and support the physical and emotional heart.

What It's For:
Hawthorn berries, leaves, and flowers are rich in flavonoids that support blood vessel tone, improve cardiac function, and reduce mild hypertension.

Ingredients:

- 2 tbsp dried hawthorn berries and/or leaf & flower
- 1 cup brandy or vodka
- Optional: 1 tbsp dried rose petals

Instructions:

1. Combine herbs and alcohol in a jar.
2. Steep for 4-6 weeks, shaking occasionally.
3. Strain and store in a dropper bottle.

How to Use:

Take 1 dropperful 1-2 times daily.

Safe for long-term use. Check with your provider if on heart medications.

172. Garlic & Olive Oil Capsules

A DIY heart-healthy supplement to support cholesterol balance and circulation.

What It's For:

Garlic reduces blood pressure and cholesterol, thins the blood, and improves circulation — especially when taken consistently.

Ingredients:

- 2-3 cloves fresh garlic, finely minced
- 2 tbsp olive oil
- Size 00 capsules
- Optional: a pinch of cayenne or turmeric

Instructions:

1. Stir garlic into olive oil and let sit for 1 hour.
2. Fill capsules using a capsule machine or by hand.
3. Store in the fridge for 2-3 days (make small batches fresh).

How to Use:

Take 1-2 capsules daily with food.

Avoid large doses before surgery or with blood thinners.

173. Hibiscus & Rosehip Blood Pressure Tea

A tart, vitamin C-rich tea to support healthy blood pressure and vascular tone.

What It's For:

Hibiscus is a well-studied herb for lowering blood pressure, while rosehips add antioxidants and anti-inflammatory benefits for arterial health.

Ingredients:

- 1 tsp dried hibiscus petals
- 1 tsp dried rosehips
- 1½ cups boiling water

Instructions:

1. Steep herbs in boiling water for 10-15 minutes.
2. Strain and sip warm or chilled.

How to Use:

Drink 1-2 cups daily to help regulate blood pressure.

Avoid large amounts during pregnancy or if prone to low blood pressure.

174. Cinnamon-Cacao Circulation Elixir

A warming, heart-healthy tonic that supports blood flow and metabolic balance.

What It's For:

Cinnamon regulates blood sugar and circulation, while cacao improves mood, supports blood vessel function, and provides natural magnesium.

Ingredients:

- 1 tsp raw cacao powder
- ½ tsp cinnamon
- 1 cup warm nut milk
- ½ tsp maca or cardamom (optional)
- 1 tsp honey or maple syrup

Instructions:

1. Warm all ingredients gently, whisk until smooth.
2. Pour into a mug and sip slowly.

How to Use:

Enjoy as a daily heart-nourishing ritual, especially in colder seasons.

175. Ginkgo-Vinegar Cardio Tonic

A tangy, circulatory-supportive infusion to promote brain and heart blood flow.

What It's For:

Ginkgo biloba improves circulation to the brain and extremities, while vinegar enhances mineral absorption and heart-supportive compounds.

Ingredients:

- 1 tbsp dried ginkgo leaf
- 1 tsp dried rosemary (optional)
- 1 cup raw apple cider vinegar

Instructions:

1. Combine herbs and vinegar in a glass jar.
2. Steep for 2-4 weeks, shaking regularly.
3. Strain and store in a dark bottle.

How to Use:

Take 1-2 tsp daily diluted in water or use in salad dressings.

Consult your practitioner before use if on blood thinners.

176. Cayenne-Cocoa Circulation Capsules

A fiery herbal capsule blend to awaken sluggish circulation and boost warmth.

What It's For:
Cayenne pepper stimulates blood flow and strengthens the heart, while cocoa supports healthy vessels and lowers stress-related inflammation.

Ingredients:

- 1 tbsp cayenne powder (start mild!)
- 1 tbsp raw cacao powder
- Optional: 1 tsp ginger or turmeric powder
- Size 00 capsules

Instructions:

1. Mix powders and fill capsules.
2. Store in a labeled jar in a cool place.

How to Use:

Take 1 capsule daily with food. Increase to 2 over time if tolerated.

Not recommended on an empty stomach or with ulcers.

177. Linden Flower Calm Heart Tea

A gentle herbal tea for emotional stress, palpitations, and anxiety-linked heart tension.

What It's For:
Linden flower calms the nervous system and soothes the emotional heart — especially useful for "overwhelm in the chest" and anxious tension.

Ingredients:

- 1 tsp dried linden flowers
- Optional: ½ tsp dried lemon balm or rose petals
- 1½ cups hot water

Instructions:

1. Steep herbs in hot water for 10 minutes.
2. Strain and sip slowly in a calm setting.

How to Use:

Drink as needed during moments of emotional stress or wind-down routines.

178. Omega-3 Herb Blend (Flax, Perilla, Chia)

A food-based, anti-inflammatory oil blend for heart, brain, and vascular health.

What It's For:

Omega-3 fatty acids help reduce arterial inflammation, balance cholesterol, and nourish cardiovascular tissue.

Ingredients:

- 2 tbsp flaxseed oil (cold-pressed)
- 1 tbsp perilla oil
- 1 tbsp chia seed oil
- Optional: 1 tsp lemon juice or rosemary extract (for preservation)

Instructions:

1. Blend oils and store in a dark, airtight glass bottle in the fridge.
2. Shake gently before use.

How to Use:

Take 1 tsp daily or drizzle over food.

Use within 4-6 weeks for freshness.

179. Motherwort Heart-Soothing Tincture

A powerful nervine for emotional overwhelm, palpitations, and heart-centered anxiety.

What It's For:

Motherwort supports both physical and emotional aspects of the heart — especially helpful during grief, PMS, menopausal transitions, or anxious restlessness.

Ingredients:

- 2 tbsp dried motherwort
- 1 cup vodka or brandy (80-100 proof)
- Optional: a pinch of rose petals or lemon balm

Instructions:

1. Combine herbs and alcohol in a jar.
2. Steep for 4 weeks, shaking often.
3. Strain and bottle.

How to Use:

Take 1 dropperful in water up to 3 times daily during times of heart-related tension or transition.

180. Beetroot & Ginger Cardio Smoothie

A vibrant, nitric oxide-boosting drink for heart health and stamina.

What It's For:
Beetroot enhances circulation and oxygen delivery, while ginger supports inflammation reduction and blood vessel health — perfect before a walk, workout, or long day.

Ingredients:

- ½ cup cooked or raw beet (or 1 tbsp beet powder)
- ½ inch fresh ginger
- ½ banana
- 1 cup orange juice or water
- Optional: handful of spinach or a squeeze of lemon

Instructions:

1. Blend all ingredients until smooth.
2. Drink immediately.

How to Use:

Enjoy 2-3 times per week as a cardio-supportive boost or gentle blood pressure aid.

MANAGING WEIGHT AND METABOLISM WITH HERBAL AIDS

Weight and metabolism aren't just about numbers — they're deeply tied to digestion, energy, hormones, stress, and how we nourish ourselves. While there's no magic herb for overnight results (and no need for shame-based "fixes"), plants can gently stimulate metabolism, support detoxification, balance blood sugar, and encourage natural energy and appetite rhythms.

This section offers teas, tonics, and food-based blends that work with the body rather than against it — helping your metabolism feel supported, not stressed. Whether you're looking to reduce sugar cravings, improve energy, or ease into a healthier rhythm, these herbs provide a grounded, natural approach to long-term vitality and balance.

181. Green Tea & Cayenne Metabolism Booster

A simple, energizing blend to stimulate thermogenesis and fat metabolism.

What It's For:
Green tea contains catechins and caffeine to gently boost metabolism, while cayenne increases circulation and thermogenic fat burning.

Ingredients:
- 1 tsp green tea leaves or 1 bag
- Pinch of cayenne pepper
- 1½ cups hot water
- Optional: lemon slice or honey

Instructions:
1. Steep green tea in hot water for 5-7 minutes.
2. Stir in cayenne and other additions.

How to Use:

Drink mid-morning or before movement.

Avoid late in the day if caffeine-sensitive.

182. Dandelion Root Detox Tea

A grounding tea to support liver function and healthy elimination.

What It's For:
Dandelion root stimulates bile production, aiding fat digestion and detoxification — both helpful in metabolic balance and weight support.

Ingredients:
- 1 tsp dried dandelion root
- 1½ cups water

Instructions:
1. Simmer root gently for 15-20 minutes.
2. Strain and enjoy warm.

How to Use:

Drink once daily, especially before meals or during seasonal resets.

183. Yerba Mate & Ginger Energy Blend

A stimulating blend to curb appetite, improve focus, and support stamina.

What It's For:

Yerba mate offers clean, sustained energy without jitters, while ginger aids digestion and increases metabolic heat.

Ingredients:

- 1 tsp dried yerba mate
- ½ tsp dried ginger
- 1½ cups hot (not boiling) water

Instructions:

1. Steep herbs for 5-10 minutes.
2. Strain and sip mindfully.

How to Use:

Use in the morning or pre-workout to enhance energy and focus.

---

184. Apple Cider Vinegar Fat-Burner Tonic

A pre-meal digestive activator that supports blood sugar and fat metabolism.

What It's For:

ACV helps regulate insulin, support fat digestion, and reduce appetite spikes — especially when taken before meals.

Ingredients:

- 1 tbsp raw apple cider vinegar
- ½ cup water
- Optional: pinch of cinnamon or splash of lemon

Instructions:

1. Mix ingredients in a glass.
2. Drink 15 minutes before meals.

How to Use:

Take before your largest meal of the day.

Rinse mouth after to protect enamel.

185. Cinnamon & Clove Blood Sugar Balancer

A warming spice blend to reduce cravings and stabilize post-meal energy dips.

What It's For:

Cinnamon improves insulin sensitivity, while clove supports digestion and reduces blood sugar spikes — great for metabolism and weight balance.

Ingredients:

- ½ tsp ground cinnamon
- ¼ tsp ground clove
- 1 cup hot water or warm plant milk
- Optional: pinch of nutmeg or honey

Instructions:

3. Whisk spices into warm liquid.
4. Let steep for a few minutes, then stir and sip.

How to Use:

Enjoy after meals or as an afternoon sweet-tooth calmer.

HERBAL ORAL CARE: NATURAL REMEDIES FOR TEETH, GUMS, AND FRESH BREATH

Oral health is deeply connected to whole-body wellness. The mouth is the gateway to the digestive tract, the respiratory system, and the bloodstream — so tending to it gently and naturally can have far-reaching benefits. Herbal oral care focuses on cleansing without harsh chemicals, soothing inflammation, and supporting the microbiome of the mouth.

This section includes tried-and-true remedies for fresh breath, gum care, minor discomfort, and even natural whitening — made from herbs and household staples you can trust. Whether you're making your own rinse, paste, or gum soother, these blends are easy to create and beautiful to use.

186. Baking Soda + Herbal Rinse

A simple, alkalizing rinse to freshen breath and reduce plaque buildup.

What It's For:
Baking soda neutralizes acids and gently polishes teeth, while herbs like mint or sage bring cleansing, antimicrobial properties.

Ingredients:
- ½ tsp baking soda
- 1 cup warm water
- 1 tsp dried peppermint or sage (or 2 drops essential oil)

Instructions:
1. Steep herbs in warm water for 10 minutes, then strain.
2. Stir in baking soda until dissolved.

How to Use:

Swish 1-2 tbsp in your mouth for 30 seconds after brushing.

Use a few times weekly to avoid over-alkalizing sensitive enamel.

187. Aloe Vera & Peppermint Gum Soother

A cooling gel for inflamed or sore gums.

What It's For:
Aloe reduces inflammation and supports healing, while peppermint cools and refreshes — perfect after flossing or dental work.

Ingredients:
- 1 tbsp pure aloe vera gel (inner fillet only)
- 1-2 drops peppermint essential oil
- Optional: ½ tsp calendula tincture or chamomile tea

Instructions:
1. Blend ingredients until smooth.
2. Store in a small glass jar in the fridge for freshness.

How to Use:

Apply a small amount to the gums with a clean finger or swab.

Use 1-2 times daily or as needed.

188. Turmeric Teeth Whitening Paste

A natural alternative to chemical whiteners that brightens gently over time.

What It's For:

Turmeric has mild astringent and antibacterial properties, helping to reduce stains and promote oral health — with a golden glow.

Ingredients:

- 1 tsp turmeric powder
- 1 tsp coconut oil
- ½ tsp baking soda (optional)

Instructions:

1. Mix into a smooth paste.
2. Store in a small jar or container with a lid.

How to Use:

Apply with a toothbrush and gently brush for 2 minutes. Rinse thoroughly. Can stain your toothbrush or sink — rinse immediately after use!

189. Chamomile-Clove Toothache Relief Rinse

A warm, soothing rinse for aching teeth or sore gums.

What It's For:

Chamomile calms inflammation and clove numbs pain — together, they bring fast, natural comfort for minor toothaches or swelling.

Ingredients:

- 1 tsp dried chamomile
- ½ tsp ground or whole cloves
- 1 cup warm water

Instructions:

1. Steep herbs for 10-15 minutes. Strain well.
2. Let cool to a warm (not hot) temperature.

How to Use:

Swish in the mouth for 30-60 seconds, especially over the affected area. Repeat 2-3 times daily.

190. Probiotic Herbal Chew Tabs

A fun, travel-friendly way to cleanse the mouth and support the oral microbiome.

What It's For:

These chewable tabs freshen breath, gently polish teeth, and introduce healthy bacteria into the oral environment.

Ingredients:

- 2 tbsp bentonite clay or baking soda
- 1 tbsp powdered spearmint or cinnamon
- 1 capsule high-quality probiotic
- 1 tsp xylitol or stevia (optional)
- A few drops of water (to form dough)

Instructions:

1. Mix dry ingredients, then add drops of water until it forms a moldable dough.
2. Roll into small pellets or press into silicone molds. Dry completely before storing.

How to Use:

Chew 1 tab daily or after meals. Store in a dry jar and use within 2 weeks.

Chapter 6

SPECIALIZED CARE FOR ALL AGES

Wellness isn't one-size-fits-all — it evolves with us. The needs of a teething baby are different from those of a hormonal teenager, a new mother, or an aging grandparent. Each stage of life brings its own rhythms, vulnerabilities, and opportunities for care. The beauty of herbalism is its adaptability — it meets us exactly where we are, offering gentle, supportive remedies that can be tailored for every age and need.

In this chapter, we'll explore herbal solutions for the whole family — with safety, simplicity, and season of life in mind. From calming colic to supporting puberty, boosting focus in school-aged kids to easing hormonal shifts, nurturing fertility to tending elder aches and memory — you'll find thoughtful, easy-to-make remedies that honor the changing needs of each body and soul.

The goal here isn't perfection. It's presence. It's learning how to meet your child, your parent, your partner — or yourself — with loving, plant-based support. You don't have to be a clinical herbalist or have years of experience. You just need the willingness to listen, observe, and offer care from a rooted, respectful place.

Throughout this chapter, you'll find age-appropriate dosages, gentle herbs, and customizable blends. Safety is emphasized — especially for infants, children, and pregnancy — and you'll be empowered to make confident choices with the right knowledge in hand.

Whether you're caring for a newborn, navigating adolescence, supporting reproductive health, or tending an elder's memory and mobility, this chapter is your guide to cultivating an herbal home that embraces every season of life — with love, clarity, and care.

WOMEN'S HEALTH: HORMONAL BALANCE AND MENSTRUAL SUPPORT

The menstrual cycle is more than a monthly event — it's a reflection of the body's inner tides, hormonal communication, and emotional flow. When in balance, it can be a powerful compass for vitality. But when disrupted, it can bring discomfort, irregularity, or deep fatigue. Herbal allies offer women of all life stages gentle support to bring ease, clarity, and balance back to their natural rhythms.

This section focuses on herbal remedies for regulating cycles, soothing PMS, easing cramps, and nourishing reproductive health. Whether you're navigating irregular periods, hormonal imbalances, or emotional shifts, these plant-based tools offer time-tested support rooted in wisdom, not quick fixes.

These remedies are gentle yet powerful — ideal for daily use, cycle syncing, or creating a nourishing moon-time ritual. You'll find teas, tinctures, oils, and food-based support designed to work with your body, not override it.

---

191. Evening Primrose Oil Capsules

A nourishing oil to support skin, mood, and hormone balance.

What It's For:
Evening primrose oil is high in gamma-linolenic acid (GLA), which helps reduce PMS, breast tenderness, and hormonal acne.

Ingredients:

- High-quality evening primrose oil capsules (1,000 mg)

How to Use:

Take 1 capsule once or twice daily with meals during the second half of your cycle (ovulation to period).

Consult a healthcare provider if taking long-term or alongside medications.

192. Raspberry Leaf Tea for Menstrual Support

A mineral-rich uterine tonic to strengthen and tone the reproductive system.

What It's For:
Raspberry leaf is rich in iron and calcium and helps ease cramping, regulate cycles, and support fertility and postpartum healing.

Ingredients:

- 1 tsp dried raspberry leaf
- 1½ cups hot water

Instructions:

1. Steep in hot water for 10-15 minutes.
2. Strain and enjoy warm.

How to Use:

Drink 1-2 cups daily throughout your cycle or during the second half (luteal phase) for menstrual support.

193. Chasteberry (Vitex) Hormone Balancing Tincture

A powerful endocrine support for cycle regulation and hormone balance.

What It's For:
Chasteberry supports the pituitary gland, helping regulate estrogen and progesterone — especially helpful for irregular cycles, PMS, or post-birth control recovery.

Ingredients:

- 2 tbsp dried chasteberries
- 1 cup vodka or brandy (80-100 proof)

Instructions:

1. Combine herbs and alcohol in a jar.
2. Steep for 4-6 weeks, shaking often.
3. Strain and store in a dropper bottle.

How to Use:

Take ½-1 dropperful each morning for 3-6 months.

Not recommended during pregnancy or when on hormonal birth control.

194. Dong Quai Root Tea for Cycle Regulation

A traditional Chinese herbal remedy to move stagnation and support flow.

What It's For:

Dong quai is often called "female ginseng" — it's warming, blood-building, and supports smooth menstrual flow and hormonal regulation.

Ingredients:

- 1 tsp sliced dried dong quai root
- 2 cups water

Instructions:

1. Simmer gently for 15-20 minutes.
2. Strain and enjoy warm.

How to Use:

Drink 1 cup daily during the follicular phase (day 1-14 of your cycle).

Avoid during pregnancy or heavy bleeding.

---

195. PMS Relief Tea Blend (Chamomile, Ginger, Licorice)

A calming, anti-inflammatory tea for cramps, bloating, and emotional ease.

What It's For:

Chamomile soothes the nervous system, ginger reduces inflammation and pain, and licorice offers hormonal and adrenal support.

Ingredients:

- 1 tsp dried chamomile
- ½ tsp dried ginger or a few fresh slices
- ½ tsp dried licorice root
- 1½ cups hot water

Instructions:

1. Steep all herbs for 10-12 minutes.
2. Strain and enjoy warm.

How to Use:

Drink up to 2 cups daily during the week before your period or at first sign of symptoms.

Avoid licorice with high blood pressure or long-term use.

196. Cramp Balm with Ginger, Clary Sage & Lavender

A warming, aromatic balm to relieve menstrual cramps and pelvic tension.

What It's For:
Ginger boosts circulation and eases pain, while clary sage and lavender relax muscles and calm emotional tension — making this balm a moon-time essential.

Ingredients:
- 2 tbsp ginger-infused oil (olive or almond)
- 1 tbsp beeswax
- 5 drops clary sage essential oil
- 5 drops lavender essential oil

Instructions:
1. Gently melt beeswax into the infused oil.
2. Remove from heat and stir in essential oils.
3. Pour into a small tin and let cool.

How to Use:

Massage into lower abdomen and lower back at the first sign of cramping or tension.

197. Hormone-Supporting Seed Cycling Mix

A simple daily ritual to support estrogen and progesterone naturally throughout your cycle.

What It's For:
Seed cycling uses specific seeds to gently support hormone balance: flax and pumpkin for the follicular phase (days 1-14), and sesame and sunflower for the luteal phase (days 15-28).

Ingredients:
- 1 tbsp freshly ground flax or pumpkin seeds (follicular phase)
- 1 tbsp freshly ground sesame or sunflower seeds (luteal phase)

Instructions:
1. Store seeds whole, grind fresh every few days.
2. Keep refrigerated once ground.

How to Use:

Add to smoothies, oatmeal, or yogurt daily throughout your cycle.

198. Rose & Schisandra Uplifting Tonic

A heart-opening, mood-balancing blend for hormonal blues or emotional overwhelm.

What It's For:
Rose calms emotional stress and supports self-love, while schisandra boosts resilience, mental clarity, and gentle detox — especially helpful in PMS or post-ovulation slump.

Ingredients:
- 1 tbsp dried rose petals
- 1 tbsp dried schisandra berries
- 1 cup boiling water or warm plant milk
- Optional: 1 tsp honey or rosewater

Instructions:
1. Steep herbs in hot water or milk for 15 minutes.
2. Strain and sip slowly, preferably in a cozy space.

How to Use:

Drink anytime emotional or hormonal stress feels overwhelming.

---

199. Menopause Hot Flash Cooling Spray

A refreshing, herb-infused mist to cool skin and calm the senses.

What It's For:
Peppermint cools, sage supports hormone balance, and lavender calms — perfect for hot flashes, night sweats, or warm climates.

Ingredients:
- 1 tsp dried sage
- ½ tsp dried peppermint
- 1 cup water
- 5 drops lavender essential oil
- 1 tsp witch hazel (optional)

Instructions:
1. Steep herbs in hot water, then strain and cool completely.
2. Add essential oil and witch hazel. Pour into a spray bottle.

How to Use:

Spritz on neck, chest, and face during hot flashes or after exercise. Store in the fridge for extra cooling.

200. Moon Cycle Elixir (Vitex, Red Clover, Licorice)

A hormone-balancing, mildly sweet elixir to support mood, cycles, and clarity.

What It's For:
Vitex regulates hormones, red clover supports estrogen balance, and licorice helps with stress and adrenal support — especially during PMS or irregular cycles.

Ingredients:
- 1 tbsp dried vitex berries
- 1 tbsp dried red clover
- ½ tbsp dried licorice root
- 1 cup brandy or vodka
- 1-2 tbsp honey or glycerin (optional)

Instructions:
1. Combine herbs and alcohol in a glass jar.
2. Steep for 4-6 weeks, shaking often.
3. Strain and add honey to taste.

How to Use:

Take ½ dropperful daily or during your luteal phase.
Avoid licorice with high blood pressure.

MEN'S HEALTH: SUPPORTING VITALITY AND STRENGTH

Men's wellness is about more than muscle mass or testosterone levels — it's about grounded vitality, balanced hormones, a clear mind, and long-term resilience. From supporting stamina and libido to easing stress and protecting prostate health, herbs offer a holistic approach that nourishes strength from the inside out.

This section brings together adaptogens, tonics, and targeted herbal blends that are especially helpful for men's unique needs — whether you're navigating energy dips, physical performance, fertility, or aging-related shifts. These remedies are rooted in balance, not extremes. They support strength, but also recovery. They energize, but they also calm.

Whether you're seeking to boost endurance, increase libido, support testosterone levels naturally, or care for the prostate with intention, this is your herbal toolkit for building strength that's sustainable, not overstimulating — rooted, not rushed.

201. Nettle Root Testosterone Tea

A grounding, mineral-rich tea to support hormone levels and vitality.

What It's For:

Nettle root may help free bound testosterone, support prostate health, and increase energy. It's deeply nourishing and strengthening for the entire system.

Ingredients:

- 1 tsp dried nettle root
- 1½ cups water

Instructions:

1. Simmer nettle root in water for 10-15 minutes.
2. Strain and sip warm or chilled.

How to Use:

Drink 1 cup daily, preferably in the morning.

202. Stress Relief Adaptogen Blend (Rhodiola, Holy Basil, Schisandra)

A calming yet energizing tonic to support stress recovery and hormonal balance.

What It's For:

Rhodiola helps combat fatigue, Holy Basil calms cortisol, and Schisandra boosts endurance and mental clarity.

Ingredients:

- 1 tsp each dried rhodiola, tulsi (holy basil), and schisandra berries
- 2 cups water

Instructions:

1. Simmer herbs in water for 15 minutes.
2. Strain and enjoy warm or over ice.

How to Use:

Drink daily during high-stress periods or seasonal transitions.

Avoid Rhodiola at night or in cases of mania or extreme anxiety.

203. Saw Palmetto Prostate Support Capsules

A convenient herbal formula to support prostate health and hormonal balance.

What It's For:
Saw palmetto is traditionally used to reduce prostate inflammation, support urinary flow, and balance DHT levels that affect hair and hormone health.

Ingredients:
- Saw palmetto powder or extract (standardized)
- Optional: pumpkin seed powder (zinc-rich)
- Empty capsules (size 00)

Instructions:
1. Fill capsules with saw palmetto and optional powders.
2. Store in an airtight jar, away from heat.

How to Use:
Take 1-2 capsules daily with meals.

Consult a practitioner if taking medications for prostate or hormones.

204. Maca Root Energy Bites

A quick snack to enhance stamina, libido, and hormone balance.

What It's For:
Maca root helps balance hormones, increase libido, and boost physical energy — making it great for workouts, stress, or intimacy.

Ingredients:
- 2 tbsp maca powder
- ¼ cup nut butter (almond or peanut)
- 2 tbsp rolled oats
- 1 tbsp honey
- 1 tbsp cacao powder (optional)

Instructions:
1. Mix ingredients until a sticky dough forms.
2. Roll into small balls and refrigerate.

How to Use:
Enjoy 1-2 bites daily as an energizing snack or pre-workout fuel.

205. Ashwagandha Strength & Stamina Tonic

A grounding adaptogenic tonic to support stress recovery, energy, and hormone balance.

What It's For:
Ashwagandha helps reduce cortisol, improve testosterone levels, and support endurance — especially helpful for fatigue and stress-related burnout.

Ingredients:

- 2 tbsp dried ashwagandha root
- 1 cup vodka or brandy
- Optional: 1 tsp cinnamon stick or cardamom

Instructions:

1. Combine herbs and alcohol in a glass jar.
2. Steep for 4 weeks, shaking often.
3. Strain and store in a dropper bottle.

How to Use:

Take ½ dropperful 1-2 times daily for 6-12 weeks.

---

206. Horny Goat Weed Tincture for Libido

A warming, energizing tonic for sexual vitality and circulation.

What It's For:
Horny goat weed (Epimedium) supports libido, stamina, and circulation — particularly useful for stress-related low drive or aging-related decline.

Ingredients:

- 2 tbsp dried horny goat weed
- 1 cup vodka or brandy
- Optional: ½ tsp cinnamon or maca powder

Instructions:

1. Combine herbs and alcohol in a jar.
2. Steep for 3-4 weeks, shaking occasionally.
3. Strain and bottle.

How to Use:

Take ½ dropperful up to twice daily for 2-4 weeks.

Avoid long-term use or use alongside erectile dysfunction medications without guidance.

207. Zinc-Rich Pumpkin Seed Elixir

A nourishing blend to support testosterone levels, prostate health, and immune resilience.

What It's For:
Pumpkin seeds are rich in zinc and phytosterols that support hormone production, sperm quality, and overall vitality.

Ingredients:
- ¼ cup raw pumpkin seeds (soaked overnight)
- 1 cup water or almond milk
- 1 tsp raw honey (optional)
- Pinch of cinnamon or vanilla (optional)

Instructions:
1. Blend all ingredients until smooth.
2. Strain if desired for a smoother texture.

How to Use:

Drink 3-4 times a week as a nourishing tonic or afternoon pick-me-up.

208. Tribulus & Ginseng Energy Booster

A powerful blend to enhance physical performance, libido, and stamina.

What It's For:
Tribulus supports testosterone production and athletic strength; ginseng boosts endurance, energy, and oxygen flow.

Ingredients:
- 1 tbsp dried tribulus powder
- 1 tbsp ginseng root powder
- 1 cup hot water or juice (for mixing)

Instructions:
1. Blend powders into liquid or add to smoothies.
2. Stir well and consume immediately.

How to Use:

Take daily in the morning or before physical activity.

Cycle use: 3-4 weeks on, 1 week off. Avoid at night.

209. Circulation Enhancer Tea (Ginkgo, Cayenne, Ginger)

A spicy, warming tea to improve blood flow, brain oxygenation, and physical performance.

What It's For:

Ginkgo improves circulation and mental clarity, cayenne boosts blood flow, and ginger warms the body and aids digestion.

Ingredients:

- 1 tsp dried ginkgo leaf
- ½ tsp fresh or dried ginger
- Pinch of cayenne
- 1½ cups boiling water

Instructions:

1. Steep ginkgo and ginger in boiling water for 10-12 minutes.
2. Add cayenne, stir, and strain.

How to Use:

Drink once daily, preferably in the morning.

Consult your provider if on blood thinners.

210. Reishi Mushroom & Cocoa Power Latte

A calming yet fortifying drink for endurance, immunity, and heart health.

What It's For:

Reishi is an adaptogen that supports long-term stamina, immunity, and emotional resilience. Cacao adds magnesium and mood support.

Ingredients:

- 1 tsp reishi mushroom powder (dual extract)
- 1 tbsp raw cacao powder
- 1 cup warm plant milk
- 1 tsp maple syrup or honey
- Pinch of cinnamon (optional)

Instructions:

1. Warm milk and whisk in powders and sweetener.
2. Blend or froth for extra creaminess.

How to Use:

Drink in the evening or during wind-down routines to build steady strength and resilience over time.

CHILDREN'S HEALTH: SAFE REMEDIES FOR LITTLE ONES

Caring for children with herbs is about simplicity, safety, and deep attentiveness. Their bodies are still developing, and their systems are more sensitive — which means the right remedy, even in small doses, can offer incredible comfort. From colic to coughs, teething to tantrums, gentle herbal care helps little ones feel better naturally — and helps caregivers feel empowered, not overwhelmed.

In this section, you'll find safe, time-tested remedies designed for babies, toddlers, and young children. Every recipe has been chosen for its mildness, effectiveness, and ease of preparation. Whether you're soothing a sore tummy, calming bedtime nerves, or easing teething discomfort, these herbal allies support children with love and care — without relying on chemicals or synthetic solutions.

Always start slow, observe closely, and when in doubt, check with a trusted pediatric practitioner — especially with babies under 6 months. You'll also find dosage tips and safety notes along the way to guide you.

Let's explore how to tend to little bodies with nature's gentlest gifts — and how herbs can become part of your family's rhythm of comfort, trust, and connection.

---

211. Calendula Rash Cream

A gentle, skin-soothing balm for diaper rash, eczema, or dry patches.

What It's For:
Calendula promotes skin healing, reduces inflammation, and protects sensitive skin — ideal for babies and toddlers.

Ingredients:
- ¼ cup calendula-infused oil (olive, almond, or coconut)
- 1 tbsp shea butter or cocoa butter
- 1 tbsp beeswax

Instructions:
1. Gently melt all ingredients together and stir well.
2. Pour into a clean tin or jar and cool until solid.

How to Use:
Apply a thin layer to clean, dry skin after diaper changes or as needed.

212. Chamomile & Fennel Colic Tea

A tummy-soothing tea to ease gas, fussiness, and digestive discomfort in infants.

What It's For:
Chamomile relaxes the nervous and digestive systems, while fennel reduces gas and bloating — perfect for colicky or gassy babies.

Ingredients:

- 1 tsp dried chamomile
- ½ tsp crushed fennel seed
- 1 cup hot water

Instructions:

1. Steep herbs in hot water for 5-10 minutes.
2. Strain well and let cool completely.

How to Use:

Give 1-2 tsp to baby using a dropper or bottle up to 3x per day. Nursing parents can also drink it to pass on benefits via breastmilk.

Not for babies under 3 months without pediatric guidance.

213. Lemon Balm Calming Syrup

A sweet, kid-friendly syrup to ease anxiety, restlessness, or bedtime fussiness.

What It's For:
Lemon balm is a gentle nervine that helps calm the nervous system and ease upset tummies — perfect for winding down at night or calming jitters.

Ingredients:

- 2 tbsp dried lemon balm
- 1 cup water
- ½ cup raw honey (or glycerin for under age 1)

Instructions:

1. Simmer lemon balm in water for 15-20 minutes.
2. Strain and stir in honey or glycerin while warm.
3. Store in the fridge in a glass jar.

How to Use:

Give ½-1 tsp as needed, up to 3x/day.

Use within 2 weeks or freeze in ice cube trays.

214. Natural Teething Gel (Clove-Free)

A gentle gel to soothe sore gums without the harshness of clove essential oil.

What It's For:

Chamomile and catnip reduce inflammation and fussiness, while aloe soothes and cools tender gums.

Ingredients:

- 1 tsp strong chamomile-catnip tea (cooled)
- 1 tsp food-grade aloe vera gel
- Optional: 1 drop vanilla extract (alcohol-free)

Instructions:

1. Brew a strong tea and let cool.
2. Mix with aloe and vanilla.
3. Store in the fridge and use within 3-5 days.

How to Use:

Apply a small amount to baby's gums with a clean finger or silicone brush.

Would you like to continue with more child-safe remedies (like Cough Soothing Syrup, Owie Spray, or Bedtime Bath Blend)? Or are we moving into 6.4 Teen Wellness, 6.4 Pregnancy & Postpartum, or Elder Herbal Care next?

215. DIY Vapor Rub for Kids (Eucalyptus Radiata)

A chest rub to ease stuffy noses and nighttime congestion — safe for little ones.

What It's For:

Eucalyptus radiata (a gentler variety), lavender, and beeswax create a calming rub for coughs and congestion without harsh menthol.

Ingredients:

- ¼ cup coconut oil
- 1 tbsp beeswax
- 3 drops eucalyptus radiata essential oil
- 3 drops lavender essential oil

Instructions:

1. Melt coconut oil and beeswax together, then stir in essential oils.
2. Pour into a small jar and let cool.

How to Use:

Rub gently on chest, back, and soles of feet before bed.

Not for use on children under 6 months. Avoid near eyes.

216. Herbal Cough Syrup (Marshmallow, Thyme, Honey_)_*

A soothing, throat-coating syrup to calm coughs and ease irritation.

What It's For:

Marshmallow root coats and soothes the throat, while thyme offers gentle antimicrobial support. Honey adds sweetness and extra immune support.

Use maple syrup for children under 1 year.

Ingredients:

- 1 tbsp dried marshmallow root
- 1 tbsp dried thyme
- 1½ cups water
- ½ cup raw honey (or maple syrup)

Instructions:

1. Simmer herbs in water for 15-20 minutes.
2. Strain and stir in honey while still warm.
3. Store in a glass jar in the fridge.

How to Use:

Give ½-1 tsp up to 3x daily during coughs or sore throats.

Use within 2 weeks.

---

217. Kid-Safe Immunity Tea (Licorice, Rosehips, Nettle)

A gentle, vitamin-rich tea for building immunity during cold & flu season.

What It's For:

Rosehips are high in vitamin C, nettle strengthens overall vitality, and licorice adds sweetness and adrenal support — safe and tasty for kids.

Ingredients:

- 1 tsp dried rosehips
- 1 tsp dried nettle
- ½ tsp dried licorice root
- 1½ cups hot water

Instructions:

1. Steep herbs for 10-12 minutes.
2. Strain and cool to lukewarm.

How to Use:

Offer ½-1 cup daily during immune season, sweetened with a little honey or juice if desired.

Avoid licorice with high blood pressure or long-term use.

218. Plantain & Lavender Bug Bite Spray

A cooling, itch-relieving spray for bites, stings, and outdoor playtime.

What It's For:
Plantain soothes itching and draws out irritants, while lavender calms inflammation and prevents infection.

Ingredients:
- 1 tbsp dried plantain leaf
- 1 tsp dried lavender
- 1 cup water
- Optional: 1 tsp witch hazel

Instructions:
1. Simmer herbs in water for 15 minutes.
2. Strain and pour into a spray bottle. Add witch hazel if using.
3. Store in the fridge.

How to Use:

Spray directly onto bites or irritated skin as needed.

219. Children's Focus Blend (Lemon Balm, Rooibos, Spearmint)

A calm-alert tea to support focus, reduce restlessness, and ease school-day stress.

What It's For:
Lemon balm promotes calm, rooibos provides antioxidants, and spearmint sharpens clarity — all caffeine-free and safe for kids.

Ingredients:
- 1 tsp dried lemon balm
- 1 tsp rooibos
- ½ tsp dried spearmint
- 1½ cups hot water

Instructions:
1. Steep herbs in hot water for 8-10 minutes.
2. Strain and serve warm or chilled.

How to Use:

Offer ½-1 cup before school or homework time for natural focus and calm.

220. Elderberry Gummy Bears

A fun, immune-boosting remedy for kids to help prevent or shorten colds and flus.

What It's For:

Elderberries are rich in antioxidants and flavonoids that support immune response. These gummies are a tasty, effective way to deliver herbal wellness to little ones.

Ingredients:

- ½ cup dried elderberries
- 2 cups water
- 2-3 tbsp raw honey (omit for babies under 1)
- 3 tbsp gelatin (or agar agar for vegan option)

Instructions:

1. Simmer elderberries in water for 30 minutes.
2. Strain and mix warm liquid with honey and gelatin.
3. Pour into silicone molds and refrigerate until set.

How to Use:

Give 1-2 gummies daily during cold and flu season. Store in fridge for up to 2 weeks.

SENIOR WELLNESS: HERBAL SUPPORT FOR AGING GRACEFULLY

Aging is not a decline — it's a transformation. With it comes wisdom, perspective, and the need for deeper nourishment. The later seasons of life call for herbs that strengthen, soothe, and protect — supporting cognition, bones, joints, heart, digestion, and spirit. Whether the goal is to ease stiffness, stay sharp, or simply feel vibrant in daily routines, herbs offer sustainable tools for graceful aging.

In this section, you'll find remedies tailored to the specific needs of elders — from anti-inflammatory supports and brain-boosting tonics to circulation teas and bone-strengthening infusions. These blends are designed to integrate seamlessly into daily rituals, offering strength without overstimulation, calm without sedation.

Whether you're caring for an aging parent or preparing for your own golden years, this chapter offers ways to nourish the body and honor the journey —

with gentle, natural care rooted in wisdom, respect, and the slow beauty of the seasons.

---

221. Turmeric & Boswellia Anti-Inflammatory Capsules

A powerful herbal combo to ease joint pain, stiffness, and chronic inflammation.

What It's For:

Turmeric reduces systemic inflammation, while boswellia supports joint function and mobility — ideal for arthritis or aging-related aches.

Ingredients:

- 2 tbsp turmeric powder
- 2 tbsp boswellia powder
- 1 tsp black pepper
- Empty capsules (size 00)

Instructions:

1. Mix powders thoroughly.
2. Fill capsules and store in a labeled jar.

How to Use:

Take 1-2 capsules daily with food for long-term inflammation support.

---

222. Ashwagandha & Lion's Mane Brain Support Tonic

A daily adaptogenic blend for memory, clarity, and stress resilience.

What It's For:

Ashwagandha calms and balances the nervous system, while lion's mane supports nerve regeneration and memory — perfect for brain fog or age-related cognitive decline.

Ingredients:

- 1 tbsp ashwagandha root powder
- 1 tbsp lion's mane mushroom powder
- 1 tsp cinnamon (optional)
- 1 cup warm nut milk or tea

Instructions:

1. Blend powders into liquid and stir until smooth.
2. Sweeten lightly if desired.

How to Use:

Drink 3-5 times per week for ongoing brain and mood support.

223. Circulation Tea (Hawthorn, Ginger, Ginkgo)

A warming, heart-supportive blend to promote blood flow and vitality.

What It's For:
Hawthorn tones the heart, ginger improves circulation, and ginkgo enhances blood flow to the brain and extremities.

Ingredients:

- 1 tsp hawthorn leaf/flower or berry
- ½ tsp dried ginger
- ½ tsp ginkgo leaf
- 1½ cups hot water

Instructions:

1. Steep herbs in hot water for 10-15 minutes.
2. Strain and sip slowly.

How to Use:

Drink once daily to support cardiovascular health and warmth.

---

224. Mobility Balm (Cayenne, Ginger, Arnica)

A topical warming balm to ease joint pain, stiffness, and muscle soreness.

What It's For:
Cayenne and ginger boost circulation and reduce pain signals, while arnica reduces swelling and soreness — great for knees, hands, or back.

Ingredients:

- ¼ cup infused oil (ginger or arnica)
- 1 tbsp beeswax
- ¼ tsp cayenne powder
- Optional: 5 drops wintergreen or eucalyptus oil

Instructions:

1. Melt beeswax into oil, stir in cayenne and essential oils.
2. Pour into a tin and let cool.

How to Use:

Massage into sore areas as needed.

Avoid broken skin and wash hands thoroughly after use.

225. Adaptogenic Vitality Drops (Schisandra, Eleuthero)

A daily energy and resilience tonic to support stamina and graceful aging.

What It's For:
Schisandra berries tone the liver and improve mental clarity, while eleuthero (Siberian ginseng) supports stamina, immunity, and stress resilience — ideal for seniors seeking gentle daily energy.

Ingredients:

- 1 tbsp dried schisandra berries
- 1 tbsp dried eleuthero root
- 1 cup vodka or brandy (80-100 proof)

Instructions:

1. Combine herbs and alcohol in a glass jar.
2. Steep for 4-6 weeks, shaking regularly.
3. Strain and store in a dropper bottle.

How to Use:

Take ½ dropperful 1-2 times daily in water or tea.

Avoid late in the day if sensitive to stimulation.

226. Digestive Bitters for Appetite & Gut Health

A gentle bitter formula to spark appetite, aid digestion, and improve nutrient absorption.

What It's For:
Bitters help activate digestive juices, ease bloating, and support liver function — especially useful for age-related loss of appetite or sluggish digestion.

Ingredients:

- 1 tsp dried orange peel
- 1 tsp gentian root or dandelion root
- ½ tsp fennel seed
- 1 cup alcohol or apple cider vinegar

Instructions:

1. Combine herbs and liquid in a glass jar.
2. Steep for 3-4 weeks, then strain.

How to Use:

Take 5-10 drops before meals to support digestion.

227. Bone-Strengthening Herbal Tea (Nettle, Horsetail, Alfalfa)

A nourishing, mineral-rich infusion for bone density, hair, nails, and overall vitality.

What It's For:

Nettle, horsetail, and alfalfa are rich in calcium, silica, and other minerals that help support strong bones and connective tissue — ideal for seniors at risk of bone loss.

Ingredients:

- 1 tsp dried nettle leaf
- 1 tsp horsetail
- 1 tsp alfalfa
- 2 cups hot water

Instructions:

1. Steep herbs in hot water for at least 15-20 minutes (or overnight for stronger infusion).
2. Strain and enjoy.

How to Use:

Drink 1-2 cups daily for ongoing bone and tissue support.

---

228. Reishi Mushroom Cardiovascular Tonic

A heart-nourishing, immune-strengthening tonic for long-term wellness.

What It's For:

Reishi supports cardiovascular health, reduces stress, and tones the immune system — ideal for seniors managing heart health or overall fatigue.

Ingredients:

- 1 tbsp reishi mushroom (sliced or powdered)
- 2 cups water
- Optional: cinnamon stick or ginger slice

Instructions:

1. Simmer reishi gently for 30-60 minutes.
2. Strain and enjoy warm or cool.

How to Use:

Drink ½-1 cup daily as a nourishing tonic.

Can also be made as a tincture for long-term use.

229. Sleep Aid Tea (Chamomile, Lemon Balm, Valerian)

A calming, sedative tea to promote restful sleep and reduce nighttime anxiety.

What It's For:

Chamomile and lemon balm relax the nervous system, while valerian supports deep, natural sleep without grogginess.

Ingredients:

- 1 tsp dried chamomile
- 1 tsp lemon balm
- ½ tsp valerian root
- 1½ cups hot water

Instructions:

1. Steep herbs in hot water for 10-15 minutes.
2. Strain and sip 30-60 minutes before bed.

How to Use:

Drink nightly to support healthy sleep patterns.
Use valerian cautiously at first — some may find it stimulating.

230. Memory Support Capsules (Bacopa, Ginkgo, Sage)

A brain-boosting capsule blend for clarity, recall, and focus.

What It's For:

Bacopa improves memory and cognitive function, ginkgo enhances blood flow to the brain, and sage supports mental clarity — a powerful trio for aging minds.

Ingredients:

- 1 tbsp bacopa powder
- 1 tbsp ginkgo powder
- 1 tsp sage leaf powder
- Empty capsules (size 00)

Instructions:

1. Blend powders and fill capsules.
2. Store in a labeled jar in a cool, dry place.

How to Use:

Take 1 capsule daily with food.

Use ginkgo cautiously with blood thinners. Consult a healthcare provider if on medications.

PREGNANCY AND POSTPARTUM: HERBAL SUPPORT FOR MOTHERS

Pregnancy and postpartum are powerful seasons — full of transformation, expansion, and vulnerability. In these times, gentle herbal allies can help support the body, soothe discomforts, and nourish the nervous system — all while honoring the changing needs of a mother's body and spirit. The key is safety, simplicity, and deep nourishment.

This section includes remedies that are safe and supportive for the unique stages of pregnancy, birth preparation, and postpartum recovery. From tonifying teas and soothing balms to iron-rich broths and healing sprays, these formulas are designed to work in harmony with the body — strengthening uterine tone, supporting mineral levels, easing inflammation, and providing comfort during breastfeeding and recovery.

Each remedy is written with care, using herbs that have a long history of safe use in pregnancy. As always, check with your midwife or healthcare provider before beginning any new regimen — especially in early pregnancy or if complications are present.

Let this chapter be a soft place to land — for mothers and mothers-to-be who want to feel held, informed, and empowered in their journey.

---

231. Red Raspberry Leaf Tea (Pregnancy Tonic)

A classic uterine tonic to support strength, tone, and readiness for labor.

What It's For:
Red raspberry leaf is rich in minerals and traditionally used to strengthen the uterus and prepare for birth — especially in the second and third trimesters.

Ingredients:
- 1-2 tsp dried red raspberry leaf
- 1½ cups hot water

Instructions:
1. Steep in hot water for 10-15 minutes.
2. Strain and enjoy warm or over ice.

How to Use:

Begin with 1 cup daily in the second trimester; increase to 2-3 cups daily in the third trimester.
Avoid in first trimester unless guided by a professional.

232. Nipple Soothing Balm (Calendula, Coconut Oil)

A gentle, baby-safe balm for dry, cracked, or irritated nipples.

What It's For:
Calendula soothes inflammation and promotes healing, while coconut oil is antimicrobial and moisturizing — safe for nursing.

Ingredients:
- 2 tbsp calendula-infused oil (olive or coconut)
- 1 tbsp coconut oil
- 1 tsp shea butter (optional)

Instructions:
1. Melt oils and shea butter together.
2. Let cool slightly and pour into a small tin.

How to Use:
Apply a thin layer to nipples after nursing. No need to wipe off before feeding unless baby is sensitive.

233. Iron-Rich Postpartum Broth (Nettle, Dandelion, Molasses)

A deeply nourishing broth to rebuild strength, blood, and minerals after birth.

What It's For:
Nettle and dandelion support iron and liver function, while molasses offers bioavailable iron and energy — essential for postpartum recovery.

Ingredients:
- 1 tbsp dried nettle
- 1 tbsp dried dandelion leaf or root
- 4 cups water
- 1 tsp blackstrap molasses (per cup, after steeping)

Instructions:
1. Simmer herbs in water for 20-30 minutes.
2. Strain and stir in molasses.

How to Use:
Sip 1-2 cups daily postpartum, especially after bleeding or fatigue.

234. Third Trimester Birth-Prep Tea (Red Raspberry Leaf, Alfalfa, Oatstraw)

A mineral-rich tea blend to nourish the body and prepare for labor.

What It's For:
This blend tones the uterus, strengthens the nervous system, and replenishes key nutrients needed for labor and recovery.

Ingredients:

- 1 tsp red raspberry leaf
- 1 tsp oatstraw
- 1 tsp alfalfa
- 2 cups hot water

Instructions:

1. Steep herbs for 15-20 minutes or longer for a stronger infusion.
2. Strain and enjoy warm or cool.

How to Use:

Drink 1-2 cups daily in the third trimester to support labor preparation and postpartum health.

235. Perineal Healing Spray (Witch Hazel, Lavender, Aloe)

A cooling, soothing spray to promote healing after birth.

What It's For:
Witch hazel reduces swelling, lavender calms tissue, and aloe soothes and hydrates — ideal for postpartum perineal care.

Ingredients:

- ½ cup witch hazel (alcohol-free)
- ¼ cup aloe vera gel or juice
- 5 drops lavender essential oil
- Optional: 1 tsp calendula tea or hydrosol

Instructions:

1. Combine all ingredients in a spray bottle. Shake well.

How to Use:

Spray onto perineal area after using the restroom or as needed. Store in the fridge for extra relief.

236. Lactation Support Tea (Fenugreek, Fennel, Goat's Rue)

A nourishing tea to boost milk supply and support digestion in both mother and baby.

What It's For:
Fenugreek and goat's rue help increase milk production, while fennel supports digestion and reduces baby's gas through breastmilk.

Ingredients:
- 1 tsp fenugreek seed
- 1 tsp fennel seed
- 1 tsp dried goat's rue
- 2 cups hot water

Instructions:
1. Crush seeds slightly and steep all herbs for 15-20 minutes.
2. Strain and sip warm.

How to Use:

Drink 1-2 cups daily as needed for milk supply support.

Avoid fenugreek if you have thyroid issues or blood sugar instability.

237. Gentle Sleep Aid for New Moms (Passionflower, Lavender)

A calming bedtime tea or tincture blend to promote deeper rest without grogginess.

What It's For:
Passionflower gently relaxes the nervous system, and lavender soothes body and mind — perfect for short windows of sleep between newborn wake-ups.

Ingredients:
- 1 tsp dried passionflower
- ½ tsp dried lavender flowers
- 1½ cups hot water

Instructions:
1. Steep herbs for 10-15 minutes.
2. Strain and sip before bed or naps.

How to Use:

Enjoy up to twice daily when rest is needed.

238. Herbal Sitz Bath (Chamomile, Comfrey, Lavender)

A soothing postpartum soak to promote perineal healing, reduce swelling, and ease discomfort.

What It's For:
Chamomile calms and reduces inflammation, comfrey supports tissue repair, and lavender adds antimicrobial, soothing comfort.

Ingredients:
- 1 tbsp dried chamomile
- 1 tbsp dried comfrey leaf
- 1 tbsp dried lavender flowers
- 4 cups boiling water

Instructions:
1. Pour boiling water over herbs and steep for 20-30 minutes.
2. Strain and add to a shallow sitz bath or peri bottle.

How to Use:

Use 1-2 times daily in the first week postpartum, or as needed for healing and relief.
Do not use if there are stitches unless approved by your care provider.

---

239. Herbal Belly Oil (Frankincense, Calendula, Sweet Almond Oil)

A calming, nourishing oil for belly massage, skin elasticity, and connection.

What It's For:
Calendula soothes the skin, frankincense supports tissue regeneration, and sweet almond oil provides hydration and softness — ideal for stretching skin or cesarean scar care.

Ingredients:
- ¼ cup calendula-infused almond oil
- 5 drops frankincense essential oil
- Optional: 5 drops neroli or lavender essential oil

Instructions:
1. Blend ingredients in a glass dropper or pump bottle.
2. Shake before use.

How to Use:

Massage gently into the belly, hips, or breasts once or twice daily.

240. Uplifting Tincture for Baby Blues (Lemon Balm, Schisandra, Rose)

A gentle mood-support blend for emotional steadiness in the early postpartum weeks.

What It's For:

Lemon balm eases anxiety, schisandra supports adrenal balance, and rose softens emotional overwhelm — ideal for weepiness or fatigue in the baby blues window.

Ingredients:

- 1 tbsp dried lemon balm
- 1 tbsp dried rose petals
- 1 tbsp dried schisandra berries
- 1 cup vodka or glycerin (for alcohol-free version)

Instructions:

1. Combine herbs and liquid in a jar.
2. Steep 4-6 weeks, shaking occasionally. Strain and store.

How to Use:

Take ½ dropperful 1-2x daily in water or tea during emotionally heavy days. Safe while breastfeeding in small, diluted doses.

Chapter 7

CULINARY AND HOUSEHOLD APPLICATIONS

Our kitchens and pantries hold some of the most powerful medicine we have. Herbs don't need to be reserved for tinctures and teas — they belong in soups, stews, oils, salts, and snacks. When we infuse our meals with intention and plant wisdom, we nourish not just the body, but the spirit and senses too.

This chapter explores simple, delicious ways to bring herbal healing into your cooking and home rituals. Whether you're sprinkling mineral-rich herbs onto roasted veggies, simmering an immune-boosting broth, or massaging a healing oil into your skin, these everyday recipes make herbal wellness feel approachable and joyful.

COOKING WITH MEDICINAL HERBS: FLAVOR MEETS WELLNESS

Herbal healing doesn't always have to come in a tea mug or tincture bottle. Sometimes, it's a pinch of rosemary in your roasted potatoes, a spoonful of turmeric ghee melting into your rice, or a warming broth with seaweed and nettles on a chilly evening. Cooking with herbs is one of the most delicious and intuitive ways to support your health — turning nourishment into ritual.

This section includes versatile, wellness-boosting pantry staples that can be made in batches and used daily. From spice blends to infused oils, these recipes are packed with flavor and function. Perfect for families, busy cooks, or anyone who wants to turn their kitchen into a mini apothecary.

241. Immunity Boosting Herb Salt (Thyme, Garlic, Sage)

A savory kitchen staple that supports immune health and adds depth to any dish.

What It's For:
Thyme and sage are antimicrobial and warming, while garlic supports immunity and digestion — making this blend perfect for cold season or everyday flavor.

Ingredients:

- ¼ cup sea salt or pink salt
- 1 tbsp dried thyme
- 1 tbsp dried sage
- 1 tbsp garlic powder or granules

Instructions:

1. Blend all ingredients in a food processor or spice grinder.
2. Store in an airtight jar.

How to Use:

Sprinkle on eggs, veggies, roasted meats, or soups. Use daily as a flavorful herbal tonic in disguise.

242. Rosemary & Garlic Infused Olive Oil

A fragrant culinary oil that boosts circulation, digestion, and immunity.

What It's For:
Rosemary improves blood flow and mental clarity, while garlic supports the immune system and enhances flavor.

Ingredients:

- 1 cup extra virgin olive oil
- 2-3 sprigs fresh rosemary or 2 tbsp dried
- 3-4 cloves garlic, lightly crushed

Instructions:

1. Warm olive oil over very low heat with herbs for 15-20 minutes (do not boil).
2. Let cool, strain (or leave herbs in), and bottle.

How to Use:

Drizzle over roasted veggies, pasta, or bread. Store in a cool, dark place and use within 2-3 weeks.

243. Anti-Inflammatory Golden Ghee (Turmeric, Ginger, Black Pepper)

A warming, medicinal fat to soothe inflammation and support digestion.

What It's For:
Turmeric and ginger are classic anti-inflammatories, while black pepper boosts turmeric absorption. Ghee helps deliver these herbs deeply into the body.

Ingredients:

- 1 cup organic ghee
- 1 tsp turmeric powder
- ½ tsp ginger powder
- ¼ tsp black pepper

Instructions:

1. Warm ghee gently over low heat.
2. Stir in spices until fully blended.
3. Pour into a glass jar and let cool.

How to Use:

Add to rice, soups, toast, or stir into herbal teas or bone broth for golden nourishment.

244. Digestive Spice Blend (Cumin, Fennel, Coriander)

A tridoshic Ayurvedic blend to support digestion, reduce bloating, and ignite digestive fire.

What It's For:
Cumin, fennel, and coriander are gentle carminatives that ease gas, stimulate bile, and balance digestive function.

Ingredients:

- 1 tbsp cumin seeds
- 1 tbsp fennel seeds
- 1 tbsp coriander seeds

Instructions:

1. Toast seeds lightly in a dry pan until aromatic.
2. Cool and grind to a coarse powder.
3. Store in a spice jar.

How to Use:

Add to lentils, rice, soups, or sprinkle on roasted veggies. Take ¼ tsp in warm water before meals to stimulate digestion.

245. Herbal Broth Bombs (Miso, Nettles, Seaweed)

A nutrient-dense, umami-rich base for soups, sauces, or sipping.

What It's For:
Nettles provide minerals, miso offers gut-friendly probiotics, and seaweed supports thyroid and detox — all in a quick broth cube.

Ingredients:
- ½ cup miso paste
- 2 tbsp powdered or finely ground nettles
- 1 tbsp ground dulse, kelp, or wakame
- Optional: garlic or mushroom powder

Instructions:
1. Mix all ingredients into a thick paste.
2. Spoon into ice cube trays and freeze.
3. Pop out and store cubes in a freezer-safe container.

How to Use:
Dissolve 1 cube in hot water for instant herbal broth, or add to soups, stews, and grains while cooking.

HERBAL INFUSIONS AND DECOCTIONS FOR HEALTHIER MEALS

Herbs don't just belong in the medicine cabinet — they belong in your pitcher, teapot, and mug. Herbal infusions and decoctions are some of the most powerful yet accessible ways to nourish the body daily. Unlike tea bags or light sips, these preparations extract deep minerals, active compounds, and flavor from your herbs — turning hydration into healing.

This section features longer-steeped infusions for mineral support, hormone balance, and cooling refreshment, plus simmered decoctions that deliver strength and immune resilience. Many of these recipes can be made in batches and kept in the fridge, offering a ready-to-sip herbal foundation for your daily wellness routine.

246. Mineral-Rich Nettle & Oatstraw Infusion

A deeply nourishing blend to support energy, hair, bones, and nervous system health.

What It's For:

Nettle is packed with iron, calcium, and chlorophyll. Oatstraw supports the nervous system and helps ease fatigue, especially helpful for depleted bodies.

Ingredients:

- 1 tbsp dried nettle leaf
- 1 tbsp dried oatstraw
- 4 cups boiling water

Instructions:

1. Place herbs in a jar. Pour in boiling water.
2. Cover and steep for 4-8 hours or overnight.
3. Strain and store in the fridge.

How to Use:

Drink 1-2 cups daily, warm or cold. Keeps for 2-3 days in the fridge.

247. Hormone-Balancing Herbal Latte (Shatavari, Maca, Cacao)

A creamy, adaptogenic drink to support hormonal harmony and mood balance.

What It's For:

Shatavari supports female reproductive health, maca boosts energy and libido, and cacao enhances mood and magnesium levels.

Ingredients:

- ½ tsp shatavari powder
- ½ tsp maca powder
- 1 tsp raw cacao powder
- 1 cup warm plant milk
- Optional: 1 tsp maple syrup or cinnamon

Instructions:

1. Whisk all ingredients into warm milk until smooth.
2. Froth or blend for a creamy finish.

How to Use:

Enjoy in the morning or as an afternoon mood lift.

248. Cold-Brewed Hibiscus & Lemongrass Elixir

A tart, citrusy cooling infusion rich in antioxidants and vitamin C.

What It's For:

Hibiscus supports healthy blood pressure and circulation, while lemongrass aids digestion and brings a refreshing zing.

Ingredients:

- 1 tbsp dried hibiscus petals
- 1 tbsp dried lemongrass
- 4 cups cold water

Instructions:

1. Combine herbs and water in a jar or pitcher.
2. Cover and refrigerate for 6-8 hours or overnight.
3. Strain and serve over ice.

How to Use:

Sip throughout the day for hydration, especially in warm weather.

249. Elderflower Lemonade Infusion

A floral, immune-supportive take on classic lemonade — delicate and uplifting.

What It's For:

Elderflower supports respiratory health and mild fevers. Combined with lemon, it creates a refreshing tonic that's also lovely for allergy season.

Ingredients:

- 1 tbsp dried elderflowers
- 2 cups hot water
- Juice of 1 lemon
- 1-2 tsp honey or maple syrup (to taste)

Instructions:

1. Steep elderflowers in hot water for 15 minutes.
2. Strain, then add lemon juice and sweetener.
3. Chill or serve over ice.

How to Use:

Enjoy on warm days or as a gentle immune tonic for the whole family.

250. Immune Chai Decoction (Astragalus, Ginger, Cinnamon)

A warming, deeply nourishing decoction to support immunity and gut health.

What It's For:

Astragalus strengthens the immune system, ginger aids digestion and circulation, and cinnamon brings warmth and antimicrobial properties.

Ingredients:

- 1 tbsp sliced astragalus root
- 1 tsp chopped fresh ginger
- 1 cinnamon stick
- 4 cups water

Instructions:

1. Simmer herbs in water for 30-45 minutes.
2. Strain and serve warm. Add milk or honey if desired.

How to Use:

Drink during colder months, at the first sign of illness, or daily as part of your immune routine.

---

251. Dandelion Root Coffee Substitute

A rich, earthy brew that supports liver function and digestion — without the caffeine crash.

What It's For:

Dandelion root stimulates bile flow and liver detox, making this a grounding and energizing alternative to coffee.

Ingredients:

- 1 tbsp roasted dandelion root
- Optional: 1 tsp roasted chicory root or cacao nibs
- 1½ cups water

Instructions:

1. Simmer herbs in water for 10-15 minutes.
2. Strain and serve warm, with milk or a splash of maple syrup if desired.

How to Use:

Enjoy in the morning or afternoon when you want a warm, bitter pick-me-up without the jitters.

252. Sleepytime Bedtime Infusion (Chamomile, Skullcap, Lavender)

A floral, nervous-system-soothing tea to wind down body and mind before rest.

What It's For:
Chamomile calms digestion and tension, skullcap soothes overactivity, and lavender promotes deep, peaceful rest.

Ingredients:
- 1 tsp dried chamomile
- ½ tsp dried skullcap
- ½ tsp dried lavender
- 1½ cups hot water

Instructions:
1. Steep herbs for 10-15 minutes.
2. Strain and sip 30-60 minutes before bed.

How to Use:

Use as part of an evening wind-down ritual to support restful, uninterrupted sleep.

253. Detox Herbal Iced Tea (Red Clover, Burdock, Lemon)

A refreshing, lymph-supportive tea for gentle cleansing and liver love.

What It's For:
Red clover helps clear skin and purify the blood, burdock root supports liver and lymph, and lemon brightens and energizes.

Ingredients:
- 1 tsp dried red clover blossoms
- 1 tsp dried burdock root
- Juice of ½ lemon
- 3 cups hot water

Instructions:
1. Steep red clover and burdock for 15-20 minutes.
2. Strain and add lemon juice. Chill before serving.

How to Use:

Drink throughout the day during seasonal cleanses or anytime your system needs a gentle reset.

254. Nourishing Pregnancy Brew (Alfalfa, Raspberry Leaf, Oatstraw)

A mineral-rich, balancing infusion to support strength, hydration, and calm during pregnancy.

What It's For:
Alfalfa and oatstraw provide essential nutrients, while raspberry leaf tones the uterus and prepares the body for birth.

Ingredients:

- 1 tsp dried alfalfa
- 1 tsp red raspberry leaf
- 1 tsp oatstraw
- 3 cups boiling water

Instructions:

1. Steep herbs in a jar for at least 4 hours or overnight for a strong infusion.
2. Strain and refrigerate.

How to Use:

Drink 1-2 cups daily during the second and third trimesters for gentle, ongoing nourishment.

As always, consult your care provider during pregnancy.

255. Brain Boost Cacao-Mint Elixir

A creamy, energizing drink for focus, creativity, and sustained mental clarity.

What It's For:
Cacao enhances mood and circulation to the brain, mint stimulates clarity, and adaptogens like lion's mane or ginseng can be added for extra sharpness.

Ingredients:

- 1 tbsp raw cacao powder
- 1 tsp dried peppermint or spearmint
- 1 cup hot plant milk or water
- Optional: ½ tsp lion's mane powder or ginseng extract
- 1 tsp honey or maple syrup (to taste)

Instructions:

1. Steep mint in hot milk or water for 5-7 minutes, then strain.
2. Whisk in cacao and any powders or sweeteners until smooth.

How to Use:

Enjoy mid-morning or before a focused work session. Can also be iced for a refreshing summer brain tonic.

ZERO WASTE PRACTICES: REDUCING YOUR ENVIRONMENTAL FOOTPRINT

Living in harmony with the earth means not only nourishing ourselves with herbs, but also reducing waste, rethinking how we consume, and honoring the full life cycle of what we use. Fortunately, herbal wisdom naturally leans toward sustainability — using whole plants, repurposing scraps, and creating long-lasting alternatives to disposable goods.

This section offers practical, herbal-inspired zero-waste swaps you can make right at home. From citrus-scented cleaners and reusable food wraps to turning herb stems into pesto, these recipes help you minimize waste, reduce your reliance on plastic and synthetics, and bring deeper mindfulness into your everyday routines.

Remember: zero waste isn't about perfection — it's about progress, intention, and creating less harm while doing more good.

---

256. Citrus-Vinegar All-Purpose Cleaner

A fresh, effective natural cleaner that puts citrus peels and vinegar to powerful use.

What It's For:
Perfect for kitchen counters, glass, sinks, and more. Antibacterial and grease-cutting, with no synthetic chemicals.

Ingredients:

- Peels from 2-3 lemons, oranges, or limes
- 1-2 cups white vinegar
- Optional: a few sprigs of rosemary, sage, or thyme

Instructions:

1. Fill a jar with citrus peels and herbs, then cover with vinegar.
2. Seal and steep for 2-3 weeks.
3. Strain and dilute 1:1 with water in a spray bottle.

How to Use:
Spray on hard surfaces and wipe clean. Avoid on porous stone like marble or granite.

257. Herbal Produce Wash (Sage, Basil, Mint)

A DIY rinse to remove residue from fruits and vegetables — using fresh or leftover herbs.

What It's For:
These herbs have natural antimicrobial properties and help lift dirt, oils, and pesticides from produce.

Ingredients:

- 1 tbsp fresh sage, basil, or mint (or a blend)
- 2 cups warm water
- 1 tbsp white vinegar
- Optional: juice of ½ lemon

Instructions:

1. Blend herbs with water, vinegar, and lemon.
2. Strain and store in a spray bottle.

How to Use:
Spray on produce, let sit for 1-2 minutes, then rinse under cold water.

---

258. Upcycled Herb-Stem Pesto

A delicious, no-waste way to use herb stems that usually get tossed.

What It's For:
Parsley, cilantro, basil, carrot tops — their stems are flavorful, full of nutrients, and perfect for pesto.

Ingredients:

- 1 cup chopped herb stems
- ¼ cup olive oil
- 2 tbsp seeds or nuts (sunflower, pumpkin, walnut)
- 1 clove garlic
- Juice of ½ lemon
- Salt to taste

Instructions:

1. Blend all ingredients until smooth.
2. Adjust oil or salt to taste.

How to Use:
Toss with pasta, spread on toast, or stir into soups and grain bowls.

259. Compostable Herbal Tea Bags

DIY tea bags made with unbleached materials that nourish both body and soil.

What It's For:

Make your own single-serve tea bags with loose herbs using compostable materials — no plastic or bleached paper.

Ingredients:

- Unbleached cotton muslin, cheesecloth, or paper tea filters
- Loose herbs of choice (e.g., chamomile, mint, rose)
- Cotton thread or natural twine

Instructions:

1. Cut fabric into small squares or use premade filters.
2. Spoon in 1-2 tsp of herbs, fold or tie shut.
3. Store in a dry jar or basket.

How to Use:

Steep like any tea bag — then compost the whole thing when finished!

260. Reusable Beeswax Wraps Infused with Pine Resin & Herbs

A sustainable alternative to plastic wrap, scented with natural plant goodness.

What It's For:

Wrap sandwiches, cover bowls, or store herbs while reducing plastic waste.

Ingredients:

- Cotton fabric squares
- 1 tbsp beeswax pellets
- 1 tsp pine resin (optional, for stickiness)
- ½ tsp jojoba oil
- Optional: dried lavender, rosemary, or lemon zest

Instructions:

1. Preheat oven to 200°F (93°C).
2. Place fabric on parchment-lined baking sheet. Sprinkle wax, resin, oil, and herbs evenly.
3. Heat for 5-8 minutes until melted, then brush to spread. Let cool and dry flat.

How to Use:

Wrap around food or containers using the warmth of your hands to mold. Wash gently with cool water and mild soap.

261. DIY Herb Dryer with Foraged Wood

A rustic, handmade tool to dry your herbs using materials from nature.

What It's For:
Drying herbs extends their life and reduces spoilage. This simple rack or hanger is made using fallen branches and string — no plastic, no waste.

Materials:

- 2-3 straight, dry branches or sticks
- Twine or natural string
- Scissors
- Optional: hooks or S-hooks for hanging

Instructions:

1. Tie sticks together in a grid or ladder shape using twine.
2. Hang bundles of herbs upside down with additional string.
3. Suspend in a dry, well-ventilated space out of direct sunlight.

How to Use:

Perfect for drying rosemary, thyme, sage, lavender, and flowers. Reuse each season.

---

262. Infused Kitchen Soap with Leftover Citrus Peels

A waste-free way to turn citrus scraps into degreasing, aromatic dish soap.

What It's For:
Citrus peels cut grease and add a fresh scent, while vinegar and castile soap create an effective natural cleanser.

Ingredients:

- Peels from 2-3 lemons, oranges, or limes
- 1 cup white vinegar
- 1 cup liquid castile soap
- Optional: sprigs of rosemary or thyme

Instructions:

1. Steep citrus peels (and optional herbs) in vinegar for 1-2 weeks.
2. Strain and combine 1:1 with castile soap. Store in a squeeze bottle.

How to Use:

Use for hand-washing dishes or surface cleaning. Shake before use.

263. Repurposed Spice Jar Herbal Toothpick Soak

A clever reuse for empty spice jars and a refreshing DIY dental aid.

What It's For:

Herbal toothpicks freshen breath, support gum health, and reuse small glass jars beautifully.

Ingredients:

- Wooden toothpicks
- ½ cup strong tea of peppermint, cinnamon, clove, or fennel
- Optional: 5 drops peppermint or myrrh essential oil
- Empty spice jar with shaker lid

Instructions:

1. Steep herbs to make a strong infusion. Cool completely.
2. Soak toothpicks in tea for 1-2 hours. Let dry fully.
3. Store in a clean spice jar for on-the-go freshness.

How to Use:

Use after meals for breath and gum support. Refill and reuse endlessly.

264. Herbal Sachets for Drawers (Lavender, Cedar, Rose)

A soothing, zero-waste scent solution using herbal leftovers or wilted petals.

What It's For:

Dried petals, leftover tea herbs, and garden trimmings can be repurposed into drawer or closet sachets that gently scent and freshen linens.

Ingredients:

- 2 tbsp dried lavender
- 2 tbsp dried rose petals
- 1 tbsp dried cedar or pine needles
- Scrap fabric squares or small muslin bags

Instructions:

1. Combine herbs in bags or wrap in tied fabric bundles.
2. Store in drawers, suitcases, or linen closets.

How to Use:

Replace or refresh every 2-3 months with new herb scraps or a drop of essential oil.

265. Garden Mulch Made with Used Infusion Herbs

A way to return spent herbs to the soil — closing the loop on your tea rituals.

What It's For:
Used herbs from infusions still have value — as mulch, compost, or garden booster. This method enriches the soil and avoids waste.

Instructions:

1. After making an infusion or decoction, let herbs cool and dry out slightly.
2. Scatter them around the base of plants, shrubs, or in garden beds.
3. Alternatively, add directly to compost.

How to Use:

Use weekly or as needed to nourish soil and honor the life cycle of your herbs.

ADAPTING RECIPES FOR DIETARY SENSITIVITIES

Everyone deserves to benefit from the power of plants — regardless of their dietary restrictions or sensitivities. Whether you're gluten-free, dairy-free, sugar-conscious, or plant-based, herbs can meet you where you are. This section focuses on adaptable, allergen-friendly recipes that don't compromise on taste or healing potential.

Each recipe here is designed to be anti-inflammatory, gut-friendly, and easy to modify. These herbal-infused foods are perfect for daily use — offering grounding nourishment that's as inclusive as it is delicious. Whether you're feeding your family, supporting a friend, or tending to your own body with extra care, these recipes make herbal wellness feel possible for all.

266. Gluten-Free Herbal Flatbread with Rosemary & Garlic

A savory, crispy flatbread that's perfect for dipping, wrapping, or snacking — no wheat required.

What It's For:
Rosemary boosts circulation and clarity, while garlic supports immunity. This flatbread makes herbs part of your everyday plate.

Ingredients:

- 1 cup chickpea or almond flour
- ½ tsp salt
- 1 tbsp olive oil
- 1 tsp dried rosemary
- 1 tsp garlic powder or 1 clove minced garlic
- ½ cup water

Instructions:

1. Mix all ingredients into a pourable batter.
2. Pour into a greased pan or baking sheet and bake at 375°F (190°C) for 15-20 minutes.
3. Slice and serve.

How to Use:

Use as a wrap, cracker, or base for dips like hummus or herbal pesto.

---

267. Vegan Immunity Soup with Astragalus & Shiitake

A nourishing, brothy soup to support immune health, digestion, and seasonal resilience.

What It's For:

Astragalus boosts long-term immunity, shiitake mushrooms offer beta-glucans for immune defense, and herbs like thyme or sage bring warmth and clarity.

Ingredients:

- 6 cups vegetable broth
- 2-3 slices dried astragalus root
- ½ cup chopped shiitake mushrooms
- 1 chopped onion
- 2 cloves garlic
- 1 tsp thyme or sage
- Optional: leafy greens or lentils

Instructions:

1. SautÃ© onion and garlic, then add mushrooms and herbs.
2. Pour in broth and astragalus slices. Simmer 30-40 minutes.
3. Remove astragalus before serving.

How to Use:

Enjoy warm during cold seasons or after illness. Freezes well.

268. Dairy-Free Herbal Butter (Coconut Oil, Basil, Oregano)

A creamy, flavorful plant-based spread to use in place of traditional butter.

What It's For:

Basil and oregano are rich in antioxidants and support digestion. Coconut oil adds healthy fats without dairy.

Ingredients:

- ½ cup coconut oil (soft, not melted)
- 1 tbsp finely chopped fresh or dried herbs
- Pinch of sea salt
- Optional: lemon zest or garlic powder

Instructions:

1. Blend all ingredients until creamy and well combined.
2. Chill in a ramekin or butter mold.

How to Use:

Spread on toast, stir into veggies, or use in savory herbal baking.

---

269. Sugar-Free Elderberry Syrup (Stevia or Monk Fruit)

A gentle immune-boosting syrup sweetened with natural, blood-sugar-friendly alternatives.

What It's For:

Elderberry helps fight viruses and inflammation, while stevia and monk fruit make it safe for sugar-free diets.

Ingredients:

- ½ cup dried elderberries
- 3 cups water
- 1 cinnamon stick
- 1 tbsp ginger slices
- ½ tsp liquid stevia OR ¼ tsp monk fruit powder

Instructions:

1. Simmer berries, cinnamon, and ginger in water for 30-40 minutes.
2. Strain and cool. Add sweetener to taste.

How to Use:

Take 1 tsp daily or every few hours at the first sign of illness.

Store in fridge for up to 2 weeks or freeze into cubes.

270. Anti-Inflammatory Herb Balls (No-Grain Snack Bites)

A no-bake, grain-free, energy-boosting herbal snack — perfect for on-the-go nourishment.

What It's For:

Turmeric, cinnamon, and adaptogenic herbs like ashwagandha support inflammation, energy, and mood — all without grains or refined sugars.

Ingredients:

- ½ cup nut or seed butter
- ¼ cup shredded coconut
- 1 tbsp ground flax or chia seeds
- 1 tsp turmeric
- ½ tsp cinnamon
- 1-2 tsp honey or maple (optional)

Instructions:

1. Mix all ingredients into a dough.
2. Roll into small balls and refrigerate.

How to Use:

Snack on 1-2 for an anti-inflammatory boost during the day. Keeps up to 1 week chilled.

---

271. Ayurvedic Kitchari with Digestive Herbs

A gentle, grounding one-pot meal perfect for cleansing, recovery, or digestive reset.

What It's For:

Kitchari combines basmati rice and mung dal for complete protein. Cumin, coriander, and ginger stoke agni (digestive fire) while being soothing.

Ingredients:

- ½ cup split yellow mung dal
- ½ cup white basmati rice
- 1 tsp ghee or coconut oil
- 1 tsp cumin seeds
- 1 tsp coriander powder
- ½ tsp turmeric
- 1 tsp grated fresh ginger

- 4 cups water
- Salt to taste

Instructions:

1. Rinse dal and rice.
2. In a pot, heat ghee and sautÃ© spices.
3. Add rice and dal. Stir, then add water.
4. Simmer gently for 30-40 minutes until soft.

How to Use:

Eat warm. Ideal during illness, postpartum, seasonal cleanses, or anytime your digestion needs a rest.

---

272. Nut-Free Basil-Chickweed Pesto

A bright, allergy-friendly twist on classic pesto — fresh, mineral-rich, and deeply nourishing.

What It's For:

Chickweed is cooling and anti-inflammatory, rich in chlorophyll and minerals. Basil brings digestive and mood support. Sunflower seeds add healthy fats and protein without nuts.

Ingredients:

- 1 cup fresh basil leaves
- 1 cup fresh chickweed (or baby spinach)
- ½ cup sunflower seeds or pumpkin seeds
- 1-2 cloves garlic
- ¼-½ cup olive oil
- Juice of ½ lemon
- Salt to taste

Instructions:

1. Blend all ingredients until smooth, adjusting oil and salt to taste.
2. Store in a jar in the fridge for up to 5 days.

How to Use:

Stir into pasta, dollop on grain bowls, spread on toast, or whisk into salad dressings.

273. Fermented Herbal Cashew Cheese (Garlic, Dill, Chives)

A tangy, probiotic-rich vegan cheese with herbal flair and creamy texture.

What It's For:
Cashews make a luscious dairy-free base. Fermentation adds gut support, while garlic, dill, and chives offer flavor, digestion, and immune perks.

Ingredients:
- 1 cup raw cashews (soaked 4-6 hours)
- 1 probiotic capsule or 2 tbsp brine from sauerkraut
- 1 tbsp chopped fresh chives
- 1 tsp dried or fresh dill
- 1 clove garlic
- Juice of ½ lemon
- Salt to taste

Instructions:
1. Blend soaked cashews with probiotic, garlic, lemon, and a splash of water until creamy.
2. Transfer to a clean jar or covered bowl. Ferment at room temp for 24-48 hours.
3. Stir in herbs and salt. Refrigerate.

How to Use:
Spread on crackers, roll into a cheese ball, or use as a creamy dip.

274. Herbal Gelatin-Free Gummies (Agar, Hibiscus, Rosehips)

A vegan, fruity gummy that's packed with vitamin C and totally gelatin-free.

What It's For:
Hibiscus and rosehips are full of antioxidants and gentle immune support. Agar-agar creates the jelly texture without animal products.

Ingredients:
- 1 tbsp dried hibiscus
- 1 tbsp dried rosehips
- 1½ cups water
- 2 tbsp maple syrup or honey
- 2 tsp agar powder

Instructions:

1. Simmer herbs in water for 10-15 minutes. Strain.
2. Return to heat and whisk in agar. Simmer 2-3 minutes.
3. Stir in sweetener. Pour into silicone molds.
4. Chill until firm.

How to Use:

Pop out and store in fridge. Snack daily for immune or skin support.

---

275. Herbal Coconut Yogurt with Probiotics

A creamy, plant-based yogurt infused with gut-soothing herbs and live cultures.

What It's For:

Coconut yogurt is cooling, dairy-free, and gut-friendly. Optional herbs like chamomile or lemon balm help calm digestion and nervous tension.

Ingredients:

- 1 can full-fat coconut milk
- 1 probiotic capsule
- Optional: 1 tsp dried chamomile or lemon balm
- Optional: vanilla, maple syrup, or citrus zest

Instructions:

1. (Optional) Steep herbs in warm coconut milk, then strain.
2. Cool to room temp. Stir in probiotic.
3. Cover with cheesecloth and ferment for 12-24 hours.
4. Refrigerate to thicken.

How to Use:

Eat plain, with fruit, or swirl in herbal honey or granola. Keeps 3-5 days in fridge.

Chapter 8

SUSTAINABLE AND HEALTHY HOME SOLUTIONS

Our homes are more than just shelters — they're ecosystems. Every product we spray, every fabric we wear, every scent we inhale becomes part of our living environment€¦ and ultimately, part of our bodies. That's why creating a healthy, sustainable home isn't just about being eco-conscious — it's a powerful act of self-care and preventative wellness.

This chapter is all about bringing intention to your everyday environment. From herbal-infused cleaning sprays and mold-fighting diffusers to natural laundry boosters and zero-waste swaps, the recipes and rituals here are designed to reduce your toxic load while reconnecting you with the beauty of simple, plant-powered living.

And the best part? You don't need to overhaul your entire house. With a few easy, affordable changes, you can begin transforming your space into a sanctuary — one that smells like lavender and citrus instead of synthetic "clean," and one that supports immunity, mood, and the health of your entire family.

We'll explore herbal allies that purify the air, fight bacteria, lift your spirits, and support sustainable rhythms in the kitchen, bathroom, laundry room, and beyond. You'll also find low-waste DIY projects and practices that support both your home and the planet — because a truly holistic life is one that heals in all directions.

So light a candle, crack a window, and let's open the door to a healthier, greener home — one remedy, recipe, and ritual at a time.

CREATING A CHEMICAL-FREE HOME CLEANING KIT

Cleaning your home shouldn't require a hazmat suit. Unfortunately, many conventional cleaning products contain harsh chemicals, synthetic fragrances, and hormone-disrupting ingredients that linger in the air and on our skin. Thankfully, herbs, essential oils, and natural pantry staples offer a safer (and beautifully scented) alternative.

In this section, you'll find powerful DIY recipes to replace common household cleaners — using antimicrobial herbs like thyme and clove, degreasers like lemon, and natural scrubbing agents like baking soda and vinegar. Each formula is designed to be effective, non-toxic, and simple enough to make with ingredients you likely already have on hand.

Start with one recipe or build your own full herbal cleaning kit over time. Either way, you'll be reducing your family's exposure to chemicals while embracing a more sustainable, nature-connected way of caring for your home.

---

276. Lavender-Baking Soda Soft Scrub for Sinks & Tubs

A gentle, non-toxic scrub to remove grime and leave surfaces sparkling.

What It's For:
Baking soda deodorizes and lifts residue. Lavender adds antimicrobial action and a calming scent — ideal for bathtubs, sinks, and stovetops.

Ingredients:

- 1 cup baking soda
- ¼ cup castile soap or water
- 10 drops lavender essential oil

Instructions:

1. Mix baking soda and liquid into a paste.
2. Stir in essential oil and store in a jar.

How to Use:

Scoop a spoonful, scrub with a sponge, and rinse clean.

277. Antibacterial Thyme & Clove Toilet Bowl Cleaner

A powerful herbal solution to kill germs and freshen the bathroom — without bleach.

What It's For:

Thyme and clove are potent antibacterials. Combined with vinegar and baking soda, they disinfect and deodorize naturally.

Ingredients:

- ½ cup baking soda
- ½ cup white vinegar
- 10 drops clove essential oil
- 10 drops thyme essential oil

Instructions:

1. Sprinkle baking soda into toilet bowl.
2. Add vinegar and essential oils. Let fizz.
3. Scrub with toilet brush and flush.

How to Use:

Use 1-2 times per week for a fresh, non-toxic clean.

278. Streak-Free Glass Cleaner with Mint & Witch Hazel

A sparkling window and mirror spray with an invigorating herbal twist.

What It's For:

Witch hazel helps dissolve grime without streaking. Mint uplifts and offers light antimicrobial benefits.

Ingredients:

- ½ cup distilled water
- ½ cup witch hazel
- 1 tsp white vinegar (optional for added shine)
- 5-10 drops peppermint essential oil

Instructions:

1. Combine all ingredients in a glass spray bottle.
2. Shake gently before use.

How to Use:

Spray on glass or mirrors and wipe with a microfiber cloth or newspaper for streak-free sparkle.

279. Citrus-Rosemary Disinfectant Wipes

Reusable herbal wipes for quick cleanups and freshening surfaces.

What It's For:

Citrus offers degreasing power, rosemary is antimicrobial, and vinegar disinfects — perfect for bathrooms, kitchen counters, and messes on the go.

Ingredients:

- ½ cup white vinegar
- ½ cup water
- Juice of ½ lemon
- 1 tbsp fresh rosemary or 1 tsp dried
- Clean rags or old T-shirt squares

Instructions:

1. Combine liquid ingredients in a jar.
2. Add cloths to soak. Store sealed.
3. Pull out and wring before use.

How to Use:

Wipe surfaces and toss cloths in the laundry. Refresh solution weekly.

280. All-Purpose Herbal Cleaning Spray (Thyme, Lemon, Vinegar)

A go-to surface spray for kitchens, bathrooms, and general household use.

What It's For:

Thyme is antimicrobial, lemon cuts grease, and vinegar disinfects — together they create a powerful, all-natural cleaner.

Ingredients:

- ½ cup white vinegar
- ½ cup distilled water
- Peels from 1 lemon
- 1 tbsp dried thyme
- Optional: 5-10 drops lemon essential oil

Instructions:

1. Steep lemon peel and thyme in vinegar for 1-2 weeks in a jar.
2. Strain, dilute 1:1 with water, and pour into a spray bottle.
3. Add essential oil if using.

How to Use:

Spray on countertops, handles, doorknobs, or tile. Wipe clean with a cloth. Avoid on natural stone like granite or marble.

HERBAL PEST REPELLENTS: KEEPING YOUR HOME CRITTER-FREE

Nature knows balance — and with a few herbal allies, so can your home. Instead of using harsh chemical sprays that harm our health and the environment, you can rely on the pest-repelling power of plants. Many herbs and essential oils are naturally unappealing to insects and critters, offering safe, effective alternatives for the entire household — pets and people included.

This section offers a toolkit of herbal repellents and deterrents you can make at home to address everything from mosquitoes and moths to ants and spiders. You'll also find gentle, non-toxic support for your four-legged family members.

These recipes are free from synthetic chemicals, safe to use around kids and pets (with guidance), and customizable based on what you have on hand. Let's work *with* nature to keep your home peaceful, pest-free, and fresh.

---

281. Mosquito-Repelling Herbal Spray (Lemongrass, Catnip, Witch Hazel)

A refreshing herbal mist that wards off mosquitoes naturally.

What It's For:
Catnip is even more effective than DEET in some studies, and lemongrass repels flying insects — making this spray both effective and uplifting.

Ingredients:

- ½ cup witch hazel
- ½ cup distilled water
- 10 drops lemongrass essential oil
- 10 drops catnip essential oil (or strong catnip tea)
- Optional: 5 drops lavender or citronella oil

Instructions:

1. Combine all ingredients in a spray bottle.
2. Shake before each use.

How to Use:

Spray on exposed skin and clothing before going outdoors. Reapply every 1-2 hours as needed.

282. Moth-Repelling Closet Sachets (Lavender, Cedar, Bay Leaf)

Fragrant herbal pouches to keep clothes fresh and moth-free.

What It's For:
Lavender and cedar repel moths naturally, while bay leaf deters other closet pests. A perfect zero-waste solution for drawers and wardrobes.

Ingredients:

- 1 tbsp dried lavender
- 1 tbsp dried cedar shavings or chips
- 2-3 dried bay leaves (crushed slightly)
- Small muslin bags or scrap fabric squares

Instructions:

1. Combine herbs in bags and tie shut.
2. Refresh every 1-2 months or add a drop of lavender essential oil.

How to Use:

Place in closets, drawers, or storage bins to keep pests (and musty odors) away.

282. Ant Deterrent Vinegar Infusion (Peppermint, Eucalyptus)

A strong-scented surface spray that keeps ants and other insects away.

What It's For:
Peppermint and eucalyptus disrupt ant scent trails and deter crawling insects — vinegar boosts effectiveness and cuts grease.

Ingredients:

- ½ cup white vinegar
- ½ cup water
- 10 drops peppermint essential oil
- 10 drops eucalyptus essential oil

Instructions:

1. Combine ingredients in a spray bottle.
2. Shake well before use.

How to Use:

Spray along baseboards, entryways, windowsills, and countertops. Avoid direct contact with pets or food surfaces.

284. Flea & Tick Herbal Powder for Pets (Neem, Rosemary, Diatomaceous Earth)

A dry, topical powder for natural parasite control on furry friends.

What It's For:
Neem repels fleas and ticks, rosemary supports skin, and diatomaceous earth damages insect exoskeletons — without harsh chemicals.

Ingredients:
- ¼ cup food-grade diatomaceous earth
- 2 tbsp neem powder
- 1 tbsp powdered rosemary
- Optional: a few drops cedarwood essential oil (for dogs only)

Instructions:
1. Mix powders thoroughly and store in a shaker jar.
2. (Optional) Add oil, then blend well and let dry before storing.

How to Use:
Lightly dust onto your pet's coat and rub in, avoiding eyes and nose. Use weekly or as needed.

Not recommended for use on cats with essential oils.

285. Spider-Repelling Cinnamon-Citrus Diffuser Blend

A warm, cozy scent that spiders dislike — perfect for fall and year-round defense.

What It's For:
Spiders dislike strong, spicy, and citrusy smells. This diffuser blend keeps them at bay while scenting your space naturally.

Ingredients:
- 5 drops cinnamon bark essential oil
- 5 drops sweet orange essential oil
- 3 drops clove or lemon essential oil
- Water or carrier base for diffuser

Instructions:
1. Add oils to your diffuser with appropriate water or base.
2. Run for 30-60 minutes near entry points or windows.

How to Use:
Diffuse daily or during spider season. Refresh blend weekly for best results.

NATURAL AIR FRESHENERS: BREATHING EASY AT HOME

The air we breathe matters. Conventional air fresheners often mask odors with synthetic fragrances that can disrupt hormones and irritate the lungs — especially in children and sensitive individuals. But nature offers an abundance of safer, more beautiful ways to scent your space.

This section invites you to freshen your home with herbs, essential oils, and plant-based elements that uplift the senses, clear the air, and support emotional balance. Whether you're simmering spices on the stove, blending a calming diffuser mix, or crafting your own incense, these recipes turn aroma into ritual — grounding, healing, and deeply sensory.

Let your home smell like what it is: a space rooted in earth, comfort, and intention.

---

286. Herbal Gel Air Fresheners (Agar, Essential Oils, Dried Herbs)

A fun, safe alternative to plug-ins or aerosol sprays — colorful, customizable, and toxin-free.

What It's For:
These small jars slowly release scent using herbal infusions and natural gelling agents — great for bathrooms, entryways, or offices.

Ingredients:

- 1 cup water
- 2 tsp agar agar powder (or 2 packets gelatin)
- 15-20 drops essential oil (e.g., lavender, lemon, pine)
- 1 tbsp dried herbs or flowers (optional)
- 1 tsp vodka (preservative)
- Small glass jars

Instructions:

3. Heat water and dissolve agar. Remove from heat.
4. Stir in essential oils, herbs, and vodka.
5. Pour into jars and let set at room temp.

How to Use:
Display with lids off in small spaces. Replace every 2-3 weeks.

287. Diffuser Blend for Calm (Lavender, Frankincense, Bergamot)

A grounding, floral-citrus blend to create peace, presence, and mental clarity.

What It's For:
Lavender calms the nervous system, frankincense deepens the breath, and bergamot eases tension — perfect for evenings, meditation, or stress relief.

Ingredients:
- 4 drops lavender essential oil
- 3 drops frankincense essential oil
- 3 drops bergamot essential oil
- Water (per your diffuser instructions)

Instructions:
1. Add oils and water to your diffuser.
2. Turn on and enjoy the shift in energy.

How to Use:

Diffuse in bedrooms, living areas, or anywhere you want to invite stillness.

---

288. DIY Room Spray (Witch Hazel, Lemon Verbena, Rosemary)

A fresh, botanical mist that clears energy and refreshes any space.

What It's For:
Lemon verbena uplifts, rosemary purifies, and witch hazel helps disperse oils. This spray works beautifully in bathrooms, bedrooms, or during home transitions.

Ingredients:
- ½ cup distilled water
- ¼ cup witch hazel
- 10 drops lemon verbena or lemon essential oil
- 10 drops rosemary essential oil
- Optional: a pinch of dried herbs or flower petals

Instructions:
1. Combine all ingredients in a spray bottle. Shake well.
2. Add optional botanicals for visual appeal.

How to Use:

Mist into the air, onto linens, or around doorways as a refreshing and cleansing ritual.

289. Simmer Potpourri with Orange, Clove & Cinnamon

A cozy stovetop blend that fills the home with warmth and nostalgia.

What It's For:

Orange lifts the mood, clove purifies, and cinnamon brings spicy sweetness — perfect for holiday gatherings, rainy days, or cozy evenings.

Ingredients:

- Peels from 1-2 oranges
- 1 tbsp whole cloves
- 2 cinnamon sticks
- 4 cups water

Instructions:

1. Add all ingredients to a pot. Simmer gently on low heat.
2. Add water as needed to keep it going.

How to Use:

Let simmer uncovered to scent your home naturally. Try variations with rosemary, star anise, or cardamom.

290. Natural Incense Sticks with Sage & Palo Santo

A hand-rolled incense blend for energy clearing and sacred atmosphere — no synthetic smoke.

What It's For:

Sage and palo santo are traditionally used for cleansing and clarity. When blended with plant resins and a base, they create beautifully slow-burning incense.

Ingredients:

- 2 tbsp finely ground dried sage
- 1 tbsp powdered palo santo wood (or essential oil blend)
- 1 tbsp makko powder (natural incense binder)
- 1-2 tbsp water
- Optional: powdered lavender, myrrh, or rose

Instructions:

1. Mix all powders and add water a little at a time to form a dough.
2. Roll into thin sticks or cones.
3. Let dry fully (2-3 days) before burning.

How to Use:

Burn on a heat-safe dish. Always use with care and ventilation.

CRAFTING HERBAL LAUNDRY SOLUTIONS FOR SENSITIVE SKIN

For many, laundry is just another chore — but for those with sensitive skin, babies, or anyone seeking a chemical-free lifestyle, it becomes a place of deep care and intention. So many conventional laundry products are filled with synthetic fragrances, dyes, and harsh surfactants that linger in fabric and irritate the skin. The good news? With just a few herbal allies and natural ingredients, you can create powerful laundry solutions that are gentle, effective, and wonderfully aromatic.

This section offers simple recipes for laundry detergent, fabric softener, dryer fresheners, and more — all crafted with sensitive skin and environmental harmony in mind. From soapnuts to calendula, you'll find herbs that not only clean but soothe and uplift. These formulas are safe for the whole family, from newborns to elders, and they help reduce your home's toxic load one cycle at a time.

Clean laundry, soft fabrics, and sweet, natural scents — all without compromise.

---

291. Lavender & Soapnut Liquid Laundry Detergent

A gentle, effective detergent that's free from sulfates and synthetic fragrance.

What It's For:
Soapnuts are natural surfactants that lift dirt without stripping fibers. Lavender offers antimicrobial support and a calming scent.

Ingredients:
- 1 cup soapnuts (or 10-12 whole berries)
- 4 cups water
- 10-15 drops lavender essential oil

Instructions:
1. Simmer soapnuts in water for 30 minutes. Let cool.
2. Strain and add essential oil. Store in a jar or bottle.

How to Use:

Use ¼-½ cup per load. Shake before each use. Keep refrigerated for up to 2 weeks or freeze in ice cubes.

292. Herbal Stain Remover Paste (Lemon, Baking Soda, Castile)

A powerful, spot-cleaning paste that tackles stains without bleach.

What It's For:
Lemon naturally lifts stains and brightens whites. Baking soda scrubs gently, and castile soap emulsifies oils.

Ingredients:
- 2 tbsp baking soda
- 1 tbsp castile soap
- Juice of ½ lemon

Instructions:
1. Mix into a paste and use immediately.

How to Use:

Apply to stains, let sit 15-30 minutes, then wash as usual. Test on delicate fabrics first.

---

293. Calendula-Infused Linen Spray

A calming, floral mist to refresh sheets, pillows, and clothing between washes.

What It's For:
Calendula soothes skin and uplifts the senses, while lavender or citrus oils add light aromatherapy.

Ingredients:
- ½ cup calendula tea or hydrosol
- ¼ cup witch hazel
- 10 drops essential oil (e.g., lavender, lemon, or geranium)

Instructions:
1. Combine ingredients in a spray bottle. Shake well.
2. Store in the fridge for added freshness.

How to Use:

Lightly mist onto linens, towels, or clothes to refresh and calm. Great before bed.

294. Wool Dryer Balls with Herbal Oils (Lemon, Tea Tree, Eucalyptus)

A reusable, eco-friendly alternative to dryer sheets — fresh-smelling and static-fighting.

What It's For:
Wool dryer balls reduce drying time, soften fabric, and carry herbal scents without synthetic chemicals.

Ingredients:
- 3-6 wool dryer balls
- 2-3 drops each of:
- Lemon essential oil
- Tea tree essential oil
- Eucalyptus essential oil

Instructions:
1. Drop essential oils onto dryer balls.
2. Let absorb for 10-15 minutes before use.

How to Use:

Toss into the dryer with wet laundry. Refresh oils every 3-5 loads.

Avoid essential oils on baby clothes or for those with severe sensitivities.

---

295. Baking Soda & Chamomile Fabric Softener

A soothing softener to reduce static, calm skin, and add a subtle floral aroma.

What It's For:
Chamomile is skin-soothing and aromatic, while baking soda softens water and lifts residues from fabrics.

Ingredients:
- ½ cup baking soda
- 1 cup strong chamomile tea (cooled)
- Optional: 1 tbsp white vinegar

Instructions:
1. Mix tea and baking soda in a large container (it may fizz).
2. Add vinegar if desired and stir well.

How to Use:

Add ¼-½ cup to the fabric softener compartment or during the rinse cycle.

ECO-FRIENDLY DISH AND SURFACE CLEANERS

The kitchen is the heart of the home — and often the first place we reach for strong soaps, sprays, and disinfectants. But many conventional dish and surface products contain artificial fragrances, foaming agents, and chemical preservatives that are harsh on hands, lungs, and waterways. Thankfully, simple herbal ingredients like citrus, vinegar, and castile soap can do the job just as well — with far less environmental and bodily impact.

This section gives you a complete, eco-conscious cleaning toolkit for your kitchen: grease-cutting dish soap, homemade dishwasher tablets, plant-based scouring powder, and more. These recipes are gentle on sensitive skin, safe for food-prep areas, and powered by herbs that clean, disinfect, and smell amazing.

Because cleaning your kitchen should feel as fresh and nourishing as cooking in it.

---

296. Herbal Dishwasher Tablets (Citrus, Borax-Free)

Simple, non-toxic tablets to keep dishes sparkling — without synthetic additives.

What It's For:
Citrus oils break down food particles, while washing soda and baking soda cut grease and fight odors. No borax needed!

Ingredients:

- 1 cup washing soda
- ½ cup baking soda
- ¼ cup citric acid
- 20 drops citrus essential oil (e.g., lemon, grapefruit)
- 2-3 tsp water (as needed)

Instructions:

1. Mix dry ingredients and essential oils in a bowl.
2. Slowly mist with water until mixture clumps slightly.
3. Press into silicone molds and let dry 24 hours. Store in a sealed container.

How to Use:
Place one tablet in dishwasher detergent compartment per load.

297. Grease-Cutting Dish Soap with Lemon & Orange Peel

A bright, effective soap that lifts grease without synthetic suds.

What It's For:
Citrus peels cut grease, remove odors, and offer antibacterial properties. Castile soap forms the base for a gentle, foamy wash.

Ingredients:

- 1 cup liquid castile soap
- 1 tbsp lemon juice
- 1 tbsp white vinegar
- 1 tbsp citrus peel-infused water or citrus essential oil (orange, lemon, or grapefruit)

Instructions:

1. Mix ingredients gently in a squirt bottle.
2. Shake before each use.

How to Use:

Apply directly to sponge or use in warm water for hand-washing dishes.

Not for use in dishwashers.

298. Castile-Based Herbal Surface Spray (Sage, Lavender)

A gentle yet effective spray that cleans and clears energy in one spritz.

What It's For:
Castile soap lifts grime, while sage and lavender are naturally antimicrobial and energetically cleansing.

Ingredients:

- 1 cup water
- 1 tbsp liquid castile soap
- 10 drops lavender essential oil
- 5 drops sage essential oil (or sage tea concentrate)

Instructions:

1. Mix all ingredients in a spray bottle. Shake gently.
2. Optional: add a pinch of dried lavender or sage for visual appeal.

How to Use:

Spray on kitchen counters, cutting boards, tables, and other surfaces. Wipe clean with a cloth.

299. Reusable Herb-Infused Kitchen Wipes (Thyme, Vinegar, Alcohol)

Quick-clean wipes that disinfect naturally and reduce waste.

What It's For:
Thyme and vinegar kill germs, and alcohol preserves the solution. These reusable wipes are perfect for quick countertop cleanups and sticky messes.

Ingredients:

- ½ cup white vinegar
- ¼ cup rubbing alcohol (or vodka)
- ½ cup water
- 10 drops thyme essential oil or a handful of dried thyme
- Cotton rags or cloth squares

Instructions:

1. Mix liquids and herbs in a jar or container.
2. Add cloths to soak. Store sealed.

How to Use:

Wipe surfaces and toss into laundry after use. Refresh solution weekly.

300. DIY Scouring Powder (Baking Soda, Rosemary, Mint)

A gritty herbal blend that tackles stuck-on messes with a fresh scent and no toxins.

What It's For:
Baking soda deodorizes and scrubs. Rosemary and mint are naturally antibacterial and invigorating to the senses.

Ingredients:

- 1 cup baking soda
- 1 tbsp finely ground dried rosemary
- 1 tbsp finely ground dried mint
- Optional: 5-10 drops peppermint or rosemary essential oil

Instructions:

1. Mix all ingredients in a jar with a shaker lid.
2. Stir or shake before each use to prevent clumping.

How to Use:

Sprinkle on sinks, stovetops, or pans. Scrub with a damp sponge and rinse clean.

Chapter 9

ADVANCED HERBAL TECHNIQUES AND CUSTOMIZATION

The lid lifts from a jar of dried rose petals, and the scent rises—faintly sweet, grounded with memory. Nearby, a handwritten blend journal lies open, stained with tea rings and pressed leaves. Three herbs are measured out on a tray: tulsi for clarity, lemon balm for calm, rose for the heart. The kettle sings softly. This is where herbalism becomes personal.

No two people respond to a remedy in exactly the same way. Body constitution, environment, season, and emotional state all shape how herbs interact with us. Personalization turns herbal practice from general to specific, from following instructions to crafting based on experience and insight. It transforms your apothecary from a shelf of jars into a responsive, living system of care.

This chapter builds on your foundational knowledge with advanced practices designed to deepen skill and creativity. You'll explore the art of blending herbs for both flavor and function, using structure and intention. You'll learn how to craft targeted formulas for specific health concerns and adapt them through the seasons. Technical skills expand as we walk through essential oil extraction and advanced infusion techniques.

We'll also draw from diverse global traditions to enrich your approach—honoring the historical roots that continue to guide herbal practice today. Finally, we'll explore how to document your process through journaling, sketching, and creating your own herbal archive.

Herbalism becomes more meaningful when it reflects your unique needs, experiences, and values. This chapter invites you into that deeper practice—where every blend is a decision, every remedy a reflection, and every formula a story waiting to be written.

CRAFTING PERSONALIZED HERBAL BLENDS

A balanced herbal blend begins before the water ever boils. It starts with intention—the desire to soothe, support, or uplift—and takes shape through a thoughtful pairing of herbs that work better together than they would alone. This is where herbalism moves from a recipe to a relationship. When you begin to craft blends based on your body, your needs, and your experience, herbal medicine becomes uniquely yours.

Herbs rarely work in isolation. Each one brings a set of actions, energetics, and flavors that can complement or enhance others. This is called synergy, and it's the guiding principle behind most effective formulas. For example, *peppermint* opens the airways and soothes tension, while *elderflower* supports the immune system and helps clear heat from the body. Together, they create a powerful respiratory tea that also tastes clean and cooling.

Blending is both science and sensory art. You're aiming for a combination that is effective but also pleasant to drink, apply, or inhale. That means paying attention to flavor as much as function. Too much bitter, and the tea is hard to finish. Too much floral, and it may overpower. Balance matters.

Start with a purpose: what is the blend meant to do? Calm the nervous system? Aid digestion? Support sleep? Once the goal is clear, choose herbs based on both their therapeutic properties and their ability to work together in harmony.

Use the Pyramid Method to create structure:

Base herbs make up the majority of the blend. These provide the primary effect and are typically mild and nutritive. Think *nettles*, *oatstraw*, or *lemon balm*. These set the foundation.

Middle herbs offer support and direction. They amplify the base or help guide the action toward a specific organ or function. *Chamomile*, *passionflower*, *fennel*, or *hawthorn* might fit here depending on the focus.

Catalyst herbs are used in smaller amounts. These often have strong flavors or activating properties that tie the blend together. *Ginger*, *cinnamon*, *licorice root*, or *cayenne* are common catalysts, bringing warmth, circulation, or cohesion to the mix.

A calming tea blend, for instance, could use *lemon balm* as the base, *chamomile* as the supporting herb, and *cinnamon* as a catalyst for warmth and flavor. Each layer serves a role, and the result is both functional and enjoyable to sip.

Start with small batches. Blend enough for one or two cups and take notes on flavor, mouthfeel, and effect. Does the tea relax you? Does it soothe digestion? Adjust quantities or switch out one herb at a time. Over time, you'll start to develop your own rhythm and palate—and your confidence will grow with every cup.

Some blends may come together intuitively. Others will need more refinement. Both experiences are valuable. Trust what you know from research, but also listen to your body. Herbalism teaches through use.

As your formulas evolve, create space to record them. Write down the name, goal, herbs used, ratios, and any personal notes. This becomes your reference for future blends and helps you learn from what works—and what doesn't.

Custom blending is an invitation to engage deeply with your body's needs and your herbs' strengths. It's where knowledge meets creativity, and it opens the door to a more responsive and meaningful herbal practice.

Blending Prompt

Create a relaxing tea blend for evenings using three herbs of your choice. Brew a single cup, take note of the taste, aroma, and how it affects your mood or sleep. Record any adjustments you'd make next time—more sweetness, less floral, longer steep, etc. This is how your herbal intuition grows.

CUSTOMIZING REMEDIES FOR SPECIFIC HEALTH CONDITIONS

Effective herbal care starts with specificity. A well-crafted remedy doesn't aim at everything—it targets a clear purpose. While general blends have value, the most powerful herbal formulations are designed with *you* in mind: your body, your patterns, your environment, and your season of life.

Creating personalized remedies begins with paying attention. Keep a dedicated wellness journal where you track recurring symptoms, sleep quality, mood changes, digestive patterns, and stress levels. Note how you respond to different herbs, foods, and seasonal changes. Over time, this becomes a personalized map for building effective formulas that evolve with your needs.

Let's walk through a few examples that demonstrate how to blend herbs based on specific health goals.

Anti-Inflammatory Daily Support

Chronic inflammation is often at the root of fatigue, joint pain, skin issues, and hormonal imbalance. A customized blend might include:

- *Turmeric root*: anti-inflammatory and antioxidant support
- *Ashwagandha*: adaptogen to reduce stress-related inflammation
- *Ginger*: circulatory stimulant and digestive aid

Formulated as a decoction or added to golden milk, this blend supports whole-body inflammation with grounding warmth. In cooler months, consider adding *cinnamon* or *clove* for additional warming action.

Sleep Support Tincture

When sleep disturbances stem from anxiety, nervous system dysregulation, or hormonal changes, layering calming herbs is more effective than relying on one alone:

- *Valerian root*: sedative and sleep-inducing
- *Passionflower*: nervous system relaxant
- *Hops*: for tension and restlessness

This tincture can be taken 30 minutes before bed. For someone sensitive to strong sedatives, reduce valerian and increase passionflower. For hot sleepers or menopausal support, add a small amount of *lemon balm* to cool and balance.

Digestive Calm Tea for Stress-Eaters

For those whose digestion reacts to emotional stress, a gentle tea can bring both gut and mind into balance:

- *Chamomile*: soothing to nerves and digestion
- *Fennel seed*: relieves bloating and cramping
- *Lemon balm*: gently uplifting and carminative

This blend works well post-meal or as an afternoon reset. In warmer months, serve chilled with a slice of fresh ginger. During colder seasons, steep with a cinnamon stick for added warmth and circulation.

Adjusting Delivery Methods

Each person's lifestyle and constitution affects how a remedy should be delivered. For acute conditions, tinctures provide fast absorption. Teas are best for daily tonics and hydration. Capsules may suit those with taste sensitivities, while salves and oils are effective for localized skin or muscle conditions.

Dosage should also reflect sensitivity, weight, and constitution. Start with lower doses and gradually increase while journaling effects. Children, elders, and those on medication may require lower doses or simplified formulations. Include breaks in chronic-use formulas to prevent overdependence or tolerance.

Seasonal Shifts

Your herbal needs will shift with the weather. Use **cooling, moistening herbs** like *hibiscus*, *mint*, and *rose* in summer to counteract heat and dehydration. In **winter**, switch to warming, circulatory herbs like *cinnamon*, *ginger*, *elecampane*, or *licorice root*. Spring calls for gentle detoxifiers like *dandelion* and *cleavers*, while autumn benefits from lung-supportive herbs like *mullein* and *thyme*.

Pay attention to your body's cues. Customization doesn't require dozens of herbs—just thoughtful combinations, tracked results, and small adjustments over time. Keep refining as your health, lifestyle, and environment evolve.

Custom Recipe Card Template

Name:
Herbs Used:
Purpose:
Dosage + Form (tea, tincture, capsule, etc.):
Adjustments Over Time:
Notes on Effectiveness:

Use this card in your herbal journal or apothecary log to track what works—and what needs tweaking. Your remedies should be as dynamic and unique as you are.

HISTORICAL AND CULTURAL PERSPECTIVES ON HERBAL PRACTICES

Herbal medicine did not begin in modern kitchens or health food stores. It was shaped in temples, forests, deserts, and villages—handed down across generations and continents. Every region cultivated its own system of healing, born from the plants available, the climate endured, and the people it served. Today's home apothecary stands on the shoulders of these ancestral traditions.

Ancient Egypt offers one of the earliest documented herbal records: the *Ebers Papyrus*, dating back to 1550 BCE. This scroll cataloged over 700 herbal remedies, including aloe vera for skin treatment and garlic for cardiovascular health. Egyptian priests, physicians, and healers used plants as part of both medical treatment and spiritual rituals, often linking botanical healing with divine favor.

In **Ayurveda**, India's ancient healing system, plants are used to restore balance among the three *doshas_—vata, pitta, and kapha. Herbs like _turmeric* and *ashwagandha* are revered for their ability to reduce inflammation, strengthen the nervous system, and support longevity. Ayurvedic medicine emphasizes constitutional type, seasonal changes, and prevention—principles that remain foundational to personalized herbal care.

Traditional Chinese Medicine (TCM) *is built on the dynamic balance of* yin and yang_—cooling and warming energies that must be harmonized for health. Herbal formulas often include five or more ingredients carefully selected to move energy, tonify organs, or clear excess. _Ginseng *is one of the most famous TCM herbs, prized for its ability to boost vitality, stamina, and immune function.*

Among **Indigenous North American** communities, herbal knowledge is passed through oral tradition, song, and direct observation. Plants are viewed not only as medicine but as relatives and teachers. *Echinacea* was widely used for infection, wounds, and immune support long before it entered mainstream herbalism. Respect, reciprocity, and gratitude are integral to Indigenous plant relationships.

African herbal systems are vast and diverse, shaped by ecosystem, lineage, and community use. In West Africa, *baobab* fruit is used for digestion and immunity. *Aloe vera*, native to parts of North and East Africa, has been used for generations to cool burns and soothe inflammation. These traditions often blend botanical knowledge with spiritual understanding and communal care.

Across all these cultures, herbal medicine reflects deep observation, adaptation, and reverence. Plants were not isolated substances—they were understood in relationship to body, spirit, and environment. Today, modern herbalists continue to learn from these systems while incorporating contemporary knowledge, safety protocols, and accessibility.

Herbalism thrives when tradition and innovation work together. A single jar of tincture or tea may contain thousands of years of inherited wisdom and a few months of personal experimentation. This blend of old and new gives herbal medicine both its depth and its relevance.

“Each herb holds a story passed down through hands, hearts, and history.”

DOCUMENTING YOUR HERBAL JOURNEY

The act of writing down your herbal experiences transforms learning into wisdom. It creates a record not only of what you’ve made, but how it worked, how it felt, and how your relationship with the plants has deepened over time. Documentation turns your apothecary into a living book—filled with formulas, reflections, experiments, and insights that grow with you.

Start with a **blend journal**. Whether handwritten or digital, it should include key details for each recipe:

- The herbs used and their ratios
- The intended purpose of the blend
- The preparation method (tea, tincture, salve, etc.)
- Dosage and frequency
- Notes on taste, scent, and texture
- Observed effects over time

Include the date, season, and any personal context—like what inspired the formula or who it was made for. These small details create depth and make the record more useful when you revisit or revise your blend in the future.

Make your journal visual. Add **sketches of herbs**, **color-coded highlights**, or **diagrams** showing layering techniques and herb categories. Draw plant parts—leaves, flowers, roots—or map out your garden layout and harvest notes. This not only reinforces learning, but also helps you track plant identification and development across seasons.

If you prefer digital tools, platforms like **Google Docs**, **Notion**, **Evernote**, or even a private **Instagram archive** make excellent visual logs. You can tag posts by symptom, herb, or preparation type and access them from anywhere. Pinterest boards are helpful for collecting visual inspiration or pinning seasonal ideas and recipes.

Photography enhances documentation, especially for those who learn visually. Take photos of your blends at every stage: harvesting, drying, blending, bottling. Use consistent backgrounds and good lighting to highlight color, texture, and detail. These images can become part of a **digital herbarium**—your own catalog of identified and used plants, labeled with dates, uses, and notes.

Visual Tip Box

- Take **macro shots** of leaves or petals to capture unique features
- Use **morning light** for clean, natural brightness
- Photograph **every stage**: fresh harvest, preparation, finished remedy
- Include labels in the frame to track batches and formulas
- Keep a folder organized by date or plant type for easy access

Over time, your records will show patterns—what works for your body, which blends you return to, and how your practice evolves. Documentation isn't just about keeping track—it's about deepening your awareness, honoring the process, and building confidence. You're not just making remedies. You're making history, one blend at a time.

REFLECTION + CHAPTER SUMMARY: BLENDING WISDOM AND INNOVATION

Herbalism thrives where creativity meets precision. Every custom blend, every experiment in extraction, every note recorded in your journal is a reflection of both art and science—intuition informed by knowledge, and knowledge made personal through practice.

This chapter invited you to take ownership of your herbal work, not only by following trusted formulas, but by learning how to craft, adapt, and refine remedies for your unique needs and the needs of those you care for. You explored the structure of herbal synergy, the depth of advanced extraction methods, and the power of cultural traditions that still guide herbalists today.

What you're building isn't just a collection of jars—it's a practice rooted in respect and creativity. You are both student and steward, honoring ancestral knowledge while innovating new expressions of healing.

Keep experimenting. Keep observing. Keep asking how your body, mind, and environment shape what you make—and how what you make is shaping you.

Your apothecary reflects more than health. It reflects care, curiosity, and commitment. Continue blending with confidence.

Reflection Prompt:

- How do your blends reflect your current needs or emotions?
- What did you learn from your most recent herbal experiment?
- What tradition or method are you curious to explore next?

CONCLUSION

Thank you for walking this path with intention, curiosity, and care. From your first herbal tea to the formulas now tucked into amber jars on your shelf, you've done more than gather knowledge—you've cultivated wisdom through practice. Every remedy you've stirred, every plant you've learned, and every page you've completed is part of something meaningful.

This book was never just about recipes or routines. It was an invitation to return to something older than instruction—a hands-on relationship with the earth and the medicine it offers. Herbalism is not a single moment of inspiration. It's a way of living that grows, one blend at a time.

As we close these pages, take a quiet moment to look around your home apothecary. Feel the shift. You're no longer just reading about natural healing—you're creating it. With every cup, every label, and every leaf gathered with intention, you've moved into a lifestyle that reflects both confidence and care. And this is only the beginning.

Throughout these chapters, you've explored the roots of herbalism—its ancient foundations across cultures, its spiritual and practical role in daily life, and its relevance in a modern world seeking simplicity and sustainability. You've built your own apothecary from the ground up, selecting tools, sourcing herbs, and designing a space that reflects your needs and values.

You've learned how to use herbs wisely and safely, how to tailor remedies with precision, and how to trust both tradition and innovation.

From teas and tinctures to balms, broths, and botanical blends, your shelves now hold more than ingredients—they hold insight, intention, and care.

This book has given you more than a collection of recipes. It has offered a framework for empowered, conscious living. Herbalism is timeless because it responds to the body, the season, and the moment. It's both ancestral and adaptable, deeply personal yet widely shared.

You now hold knowledge that supports wellness, nurtures the earth, and connects you to a global lineage of home healers. That power is yours to carry forward.

Herbal living creates real, lasting shifts. You notice changes in your health—fewer chemicals, fewer side effects, and remedies that respond to your unique body and needs. You're no longer reaching for a quick fix but supporting long-term wellness with intention.

Your home becomes cleaner, your choices more sustainable. Each salve, spray, or tea you craft replaces something synthetic, reducing your impact on the earth while deepening your relationship with it.

Financially, the benefits grow too. Homemade remedies lower your reliance on expensive over-the-counter products and empower you to care for your household naturally.

This is more than healing—it's stewardship. A mindful way of living that supports body, home, and planet with wisdom and care.

Keep going. Every blend you create, every herb you grow, every note you scribble into your journal adds to your knowledge and deepens your practice. Herbalism thrives through experimentation—try new combinations, adjust your methods, and pay attention to what works for you.

Read more. Connect with herbal communities. Take a class. There's always more to discover, and you don't have to do it alone.

Stay curious. Stay grounded. Let your intuition guide you as much as your books do. There's no single right way—only your way, refined through time and attention.

Start a garden, however small. Share a remedy with someone you love. These are the moments where herbalism becomes real—and deeply yours.

Most evenings, I brew rose and tulsi tea as the light begins to fade. It's a quiet ritual—nothing dramatic, just a moment to return to myself. There was a time I reached for noise, for speed, for quick relief. Now, I reach for herbs. One cup at a time, they've helped me soften, slow down, and listen—both to my body and to the world around me.

Herbs didn't just support my health—they reshaped my relationship with care. They reminded me that healing is often found in small, consistent acts. And that nature always meets us when we meet it with respect.

You're part of something bigger—a quiet, powerful revival of homegrown healing and natural wisdom. Every time you reach for a jar of herbs, you join a global community of caregivers, growers, and healers. You're not doing this alone.

The plants are with you. So are we.

Together, we're remembering how to heal—with our hands, our hearts, and the wild wisdom of the earth.

REFERENCES

- *Apothecary* https://en.wikipedia.org/wiki/Apothecary
- *Herbal versus synthetic drugs; beliefs and facts - PMC* https://pmc.ncbi.nlm.nih.gov/articles/PMC5297475/#:~:text=Synthetic%20drugs%20address%20symptoms%20caused,the%20body's%20own%20healing%20process.
- *Ayurveda and Traditional Chinese Medicine* https://pmc.ncbi.nlm.nih.gov/articles/PMC1297513/
- *Historic Medicines and Cure-alls in America* https://www.ohsu.edu/historical-collections-archives/theres-cure-historic-medicines-and-cure-alls-america
- *Essential Tools for Your Home Apothecary - Calhoun Farm* https://calhounfarmstead.com/blogs/news/essential-tools-for-your-home-apothecary
- *4 Bulk Herb Wholesalers You Can Trust* https://www.motherearthliving.com/health-and-wellness/bulk-herb-wholesalers-you-can-trust-zmez16jazolc/
- *Indoor vs. Outdoor Growing: Benefits and Drawbacks* https://medicgrow.com/blogs/general-tips/indoor-vs-outdoor-growing-benefits-and-drawbacks?srsltid=AfmBOorhMUGWI7RRqQrXUioESMQAM7tf1t3gt-iNMbLrgE9HBcweMbHe
- *Legalities of Herbal Products Businesses in the United States* https://chestnutherbs.com/legalities-of-herbal-products-businesses-in-the-united-states/

- *WHO guidelines on safety monitoring of herbal medicines ...* https://apps.who.int/iris/bitstream/handle/10665/43034/9241592214_eng.pdf
- *Herbal Medicine Dosage Standardisation* https://www.sciencedirect.com/science/article/abs/pii/S2210803324000460
- *Identification of medicinal herbs in Asteraceae and ...* https://www.sciencedirect.com/science/article/abs/pii/S2210803321000920
- *Herb–Drug Interactions: Worlds Intersect with the Patient at ...* https://pmc.ncbi.nlm.nih.gov/articles/PMC8401017/
- *YOUR HERBAL FIRST Aid Kit Needs These 15 Plants* https://animamundiherbals.com/blogs/blog/your-herbal-first-aid-kit-needs-these-15-plants?srsltid=AfmBOop_tm7NcKjIuNbHIxNAEeCEDy-E3K8LNvB_2tHq6autseZWGcQf
- *Natural Ingredients to Improve Immunity - PMC* https://pmc.ncbi.nlm.nih.gov/articles/PMC10143734/
- *10 Healthy Herbal Teas You Should Try* https://www.healthline.com/nutrition/10-herbal-teas
- *Natural Remedies to Alleviate Anxiety* https://www.webmd.com/anxiety-panic/natural-remedies-for-anxiety
- *12 of the Best Herbs for Skin Care and How to Use Them* https://bhskin.com/blog/12-best-herbal-skincare-products-2022/
- *Home Remedies for Hair Growth: Natural Solutions* https://www.verywellhealth.com/home-remedies-for-hair-growth-8599227
- *Neuroprotective Herbs for the Management of Alzheimer's ...* https://pmc.ncbi.nlm.nih.gov/articles/PMC8068256/

- *The 10 Best Herbs for Liver Health: Benefits and Precautions* https://www.healthline.com/nutrition/herbs-for-liver
- *5 Impressive Herbs That Help Balance your Hormones* https://www.healthline.com/nutrition/herbs-that-balance-hormones
- *6 Natural Remedies for Enlarged Prostate (BPH)* https://www.healthline.com/health/enlarged-prostate/natural-remedies
- *A Guide to Common Medicinal Herbs* https://www.nationwidechildrens.org/family-resources-education/family-resources-library/a-guide-to-common-medicinal-herbs
- *How to Use Natural & Herbal Remedies to Bolster Senior Health* https://www.seniorlifestyle.com/resources/blog/natural-herbal-remedies-senior-health/
- *Culinary Herbs and Spices: Their Bioactive Properties, the ...* https://pmc.ncbi.nlm.nih.gov/articles/PMC4227268/
- *Infusions & Decoctions* https://grassrootsremedies.co.uk/wp-content/uploads/2021/06/Infusions-Decoctions-copy.pdf
- *Mastering a Zero-Waste Kitchen: Tips and Hacks for ...* https://www.irkmagazine.com/post/mastering-a-zero-waste-kitchen-tips-and-hacks-for-sustainable-cooking
- *How to Adapt Recipes for Dietary Restrictions* https://www.escoffier.edu/blog/recipes/how-to-adapt-recipes-for-dietary-restrictions/
- *Identifying Greener Cleaning Products | US EPA* https://www.epa.gov/greenerproducts/identifying-greener-cleaning-products
- *8 Natural & Homemade Insecticides: Save Your Garden ...* https://www.treehugger.com/natural-homemade-insecticides-save-your-garden-without-killing-earth-4858819

- *10 Best Homemade Air Freshener Recipes* https://www.theprairiehomestead.com/2013/06/homemade-air-fresheners.html
- *How to Choose a Sensitive Skin Detergent* https://www.all-laundry.com/sensitive-skin/selecting-a-sensitive-skin-detergent.html
- *How to Make Your Own Tea Blends: The Pyramid Method* https://www.growcreatesip.com/blog/how-to-make-your-own-tea-blends-the-pyramid-method
- *Supercritical Carbon Dioxide Extraction of Four Medicinal ...* https://pmc.ncbi.nlm.nih.gov/articles/PMC8468049/
- *Ebers Papyrus* https://en.wikipedia.org/wiki/Ebers_Papyrus
- *How to Create Your Own Herbal Materia Medica https://bloominstitute.ca/how-to-create-your-own-herbal-materia-medica/*

Made in the USA
Monee, IL
04 November 2026

67384053R00138